14-120-815

THE
AGELESS
WOMAN

THE
AGELESS
WOMAN

*Menopause, Hormones, and the Quest
for Youth*

❦

Sherwin A. Kaufman, M.D.

Prentice-Hall, Inc.
Englewood Cliffs, New Jersey

To those I love—
my wife, Claire,
and my sons,
Kenneth, Keith, and Michael

I wish to thank

The many patients whose searching questions have indicated the need for this book. *My wife, Claire,* the first to see each chapter as it was completed, for her sensitive, perceptive comments and gentle encouragement. *Ann Pinchot,* for editorial assistance with the final draft. *Dr. Martin J. Clyman, Dr. S. Leon Israel,* and *Dr. Somers H. Sturgis* for taking the time from their busy schedules to read the book in manuscript. Their warm, personal interest is deeply appreciated.

Foreword

The Ageless Woman is an important book. It is a well-documented, common-sense answer to the confusion in lay articles concerning hormones, cancer and bodily changes. It includes what every woman should know about herself and is written in terms that she can understand. Among the many examples from Dr. Kaufman's own practice, she may well respond with "but that's what I had always thought" or "this is exactly what's happening to me!" As she reads further, she learns that there are, to be sure, differences of medical opinion. But she is an individual and must be treated as such.

Estrogen is the theme of the book—its benefits and limitations. But Dr. Kaufman discusses hormones in the context of the whole range of problems of womanhood—social and marital difficulties, the universal quest for ageless beauty, factors that may contribute to depression, and much more.

There are many golden nuggets that enrich each chapter. Myths, historical and literary data, false theories and quack remedies of the past enhance the discussion of ideas about the present. It is fascinating to note the ancient superstitions that were believed to offer a longer life. To quote Dr. Kaufman, "It is hardly surprising that the current speculation about hormones to remain young . . . and slow down the aging process seems to have reawakened woman's dream to be forever attractive, forever young."

The author's own philosophy and the theories of others are

Foreword

abundantly documented by a pertinent bibliography that includes references from Socrates to Shakespeare. Their appropriateness bears witness to the wisdom and wide experience with which Dr. Kaufman has painted his thoughtful and candid portrait of the "ageless woman."

Somers H. Sturgis, M.D.
Clinical Professor of Gynecology,
Harvard Medical School

Contents

THE
AGELESS
WOMAN

1

Longevity and the Quest
for Youth and Beauty

*No man can have a peaceful life who
thinks too much of lengthening it*
SENECA

The desire to prolong life and to postpone aging is as old as
history.

The Book of Genesis describes two trees in the Gar-
den of Eden, the Tree of Knowledge and the Tree of Life.
Adam did taste of the first tree, and he became wise. But
he was driven out of Eden that he might not taste of the
other and live forever.

Among primitives, careful observance of rituals and
divine omens were probably the most common means of
seeking a long life. The Chippewa tribe believed that at
critical times in one's life a guardian spirit would appear.
To heed the warnings of this spirit was a way to achieve a
long life. The Ainu prayed to their dead for longevity. The
Maori believed that obedience to their own priests was the
key to longevity. The ancient Hebrews admonished:
"Honor thy mother and thy father, that thy days be long in
the land. . . ." Modern prayers often contain similar peti-
tions.

Australian primitive tribal cultures had some novel
ideas on longevity. The Berbers believed that those who led
good moral and truthful lives would live the longest. The

1

Dieri claimed that "a man could escape gray hair by properly avoiding his mother-in-law."

Certain fetish objects or words thought to have a magic significance were also used to forestall old age. Yukaghir women believed that keeping vermin on their bodies would prolong life. Crow women kept a special rattle to help preserve their bodies; the Kwakiutl bathed in urine. The Samoans counted on the ava root to aid their quest for a long life. The Xosa advised the removal of gray hairs. And a Hottentot who sneezed would repeat the magic words, "Live to an old age."

In short, no one *wants* to grow old. There's a story about W. Somerset Maugham at his eightieth birthday party at the Garrick Club. He acknowledged a standing ovation with the words, "There are many virtues in growing old." An embarrassingly long pause followed, and the audience was becoming uneasy. He looked up and continued, "I'm just . . . trying . . . to think what they are!"

Maugham was not the only famous person to remain vital and productive well into old age. There are many others—Churchill, Toscanini, Chagall, Casals. Most of us may be unaware that in the 1960 census there were over 10,000 Americans 100 years or older; one for every 17,000 persons. Probably the oldest living man on earth is Shirali Muslimov, a Russian peasant farmer who claims to be 161 years old! (Without proper authentication this, of course, may be questioned.) Biologically the maximum life span for humans is about 115 years. If that seems long, think of the Galápagos tortoise with its life span of 176 years. The longevity of mammals or reptiles is dwarfed completely beside that of such trees as the giant sequoia—3,000 years— or the oldest of *all* living things, the bristlecone pine— 4,600 years.

Consider the human life span. We start to age the

2

moment of conception! Even at birth the umbilical cord is already "aged" and is no longer needed. Man begins "dying," so to speak, the day he is born.

What causes aging?

There's a popular saying that if you want to live long, pick your ancestors wisely. In other words, if your parents had long lives and their parents before them did, chances are you will. We have all known people who look much younger than their years and never seem to age.

This can be embarrassing. A perpetually young-looking surgeon told me that a few of his patients have remarked, "What a coincidence. I was operated on by your father about 25 years ago. You certainly resemble him." He acknowledges this with a nod, and when he leaves the patient's room, says to his entourage, "I operated on her, but I've stopped trying to explain!"

Very convincing evidence for the influence of heredity on longevity is that, while identical twins live to almost the same age, the life span of fraternal twins varies greatly. Of interest too is a disease called progeria. In this disorder there is an accelerated aging process in which hardening of the arteries and wrinkling of the skin begin at about age seven. The average age of death in progeria is sixteen years, generally from coronary disease.

Aging is also influenced by environmental factors. An obvious example is the extended life span of animals in captivity, which far exceeds their life span in the wild where they are in danger of starvation, disease or slaughter. Environmental extremes have a similar effect on humans. For example, people can survive in extreme climates. But a price is paid. Such people tend to have shorter lives than those who live in temperate climates. No great civilization has ever arisen in the frigid zones. Tropical temperatures tend to be debilitating, and abrupt seasonal changes may impose a strain on the cardiovascular system.

The women of certain African tribes begin to age very

3

early. A Gabun Negress of twenty may seem like an old woman. Shangella women of the same age are often wrinkled and have lost their ability to conceive. These features vary from tribe to tribe. Aging in such instances is attributed mainly to the hard life they lead.

On the other hand, the isolated African Mabaans seem to have an unusually slow aging process, with low blood pressure, no known coronary disease and measurably superior hearing as determined by air-bone gap tests. Whether their low cholesterol diets, active lives and abstinence from smoking play a role—is it nature or nurture?—or other factors, requires further research.

A *short* life span is the fate of the teeming populations of countries such as India and China. This shorter life expectancy is not because their aging process is any faster than our own, but because of environmental factors—contagious diseases, poor nutrition, frequent childbearing among women. It is because of environmental improvement that worldwide life expectancy rose from only 25 years at the beginning of the Christian era to a little less than 50 by 1900. Today a boy baby born in the United States can expect to live to about 70, a girl to almost 80.

As we know, overweight, heavy smoking, and air pollution tend to shorten the life span. Even a person's marital state plays a role. Statistically, married people live longer than those who are single, widowed or divorced (one spouse tends to take care of the other). Country people generally live longer than city dwellers. And women now outlive men—in fact, the female outlives the male in practically every known species.

One of the most fascinating fields of research involves not hereditary or environmental influences on aging, but rather *biological* ones. It seems that even under the most ideal circumstances, aging proceeds according to a specific genetically determined time-clock schedule for each species. It's true that the average American lives much longer

4

than he did a century ago. But the *maximum* life span has not changed at all. It never has.

Because we have been able to decrease death rates for younger age groups, more and more people now live to old age. But no "older" than granny several generations back. It has not been possible to decrease death rates significantly among the elderly, apparently because at this age deterioration sets in; and if you avoid one disease, chances are another will strike. It has been estimated that if a way to eliminate cancer were found, only 1.5 years would be added to the average life span. Even if all cardiovascular and kidney diseases were eliminated, the average life span might be increased by only 7.5 years. The death rate from all causes increases exponentially with age.

This biological time-clock schedule appears to be true of all mammals. For example, mice that have been kept all their lives in a completely germ-free environment do not live any longer than others raised under just reasonable sanitary conditions.

Death is not part of the genetic program of certain other species, such as bacteria and trees. Under optimal conditions, a suspension of bacteria might be called "immortal"—never really dying. The aging of trees is also unique. A seed from a 3,000-year-old giant sequoia tree is as good as one from a young tree. In short, under optimal conditions old trees never die. What happens, though, is that growth in terrain is never really ideal, and so trees age and die because of mechanical difficulties.

Several interesting biological theories of the aging mechanism have been proposed. One is the wear-and-tear theory, which originally proposed that each person has an energy quota. Others have postulated a life span proportional to metabolic energy expenditure. That is, if faster metabolism is forced, a cell's ribonucleic acid (RNA) is used up sooner and it may therefore age faster. Another theory suggests that aging is the total wear and tear (that

5

is, stress) to which the body has been exposed, or the amount of disease to which the person has been subjected. The waste product theory proposes that senile pigments accumulate in cells and contribute to aging. The collagen theory states that collagen, a fibrous protein, gradually shrinks and harms the tissue of which it forms a part. And the calcium theory proposes that aging is due to a calcium shift from bone to soft tissue.

The somatic mutation theory suggests a relationship between aging and chromosome aberrations or mutations. The mutations may occur spontaneously, perpetuated by subsequent cell divisions. But since there is a long time lag between the mutation and the effect on aging, only mutations produced while the organism is relatively young will shorten life span. Since many mutations are considered harmful, the cells gradually lose their ability to perform vital functions. Such mutations may lead to allergic disorders within the body by manufacturing proteins not identical to the original proteins. Or, perhaps, they may lead to circulatory failure by lining the blood vessels.

Another theory is the hormonal one. When hormones were first discovered, they were thought to cause aging. Since the pituitary master gland influences the sex glands and helps regulate growth and maturity, it was natural to assume the glandular mechanism also determined longevity. But after much research, such a connection has not been established, and efforts to restore youth through various hormones have failed. Of the many hormones in the body, some increase secretion with age, some decrease, some remain unchanged, and some simply fluctuate.

As might be expected, particular attention has been given to gonadal or sex hormones—such as estrogen in women—as a clue to aging. But evidence to date indicates that this hormone does not affect life span. Actually, its decrease during later years seems a symptom rather than a cause of aging. That is, aging is not due to lack of estrogen.

6

A woman ages appreciably between puberty and menopause, during which time she certainly has, by any standards, adequate amounts of estrogen.

Sir George White Pickering thought it "odd that a creature so complex and so beautifully fashioned as man should have to die, particularly when he has perhaps spent a lifetime in acquiring knowledge and wisdom, in perfecting nature's finest instrument—the human mind." It does seem strange. And throughout history man has attempted to reverse aging, to prolong life, to conquer death. So far, unsuccessfully.

To conquer death, it is first necessary to unravel the secret of life. The most exciting progress in this direction has been through the discovery of the basic building blocks of individual cells. Like the power of an unleashed atom, the amount of life-activity in a single cell is phenomenal. The more than 3 billion people now living on earth arose from twice as many gametes (6 billion), the total volume of which is no larger than the size of a raindrop; this incredibly small amount contains all the genetic information which the human race has received!

The basic unit of heredity in every form of life is composed of spiral strands of protein material called DNA, which is transcribed to "messenger-molecules" called RNA. Further research may someday teach us how to make DNA and RNA duplicate themselves, which would provide clues to the origins of life.

But living longer apparently isn't enough. Along with the quest for longevity is the search for youth. Bob Hope's secret for staying young, he says, is lying about his age. This is an easy way to stop the clock, and even turn it back.

This wish to reverse the aging process dates back to ancient lore. In a Norse myth the goddess Idhunk kept magic apples in a special chest. The aging gods ate them to regain their youthful powers. According to Navaho Indian legend, an old woman could become young again by passing back and forth through a door which faced the north. Another tribe, the Haida, told of a great magician who had the power of making the aged spry again simply by spitting powerful medicine over their wrinkled skin. The primitive Yukaghir of Siberia believed there was "an old woman who once possessed the 'water of youth' which could change the most decrepit matron back to a spry young maiden." But the water was lost.

The Trobrianders had legends of the past, describing how people could rejuvenate themselves simply by shedding their skins. The art was said to be lost through the carelessness of a certain ancestor. And the Semang had a vision of "a land beyond the setting sun where men grew old and young again, and never had to die."

It was Indian legend, too, which in 1512 prompted Juan Ponce de León to seek the "Fountain of Perpetual Youth". Some Indians told him that such a fountain did exist. At the time he was 52 years old and in poor health. He never found the elusive fountain—but he did discover Florida, where he lived (without benefit of magic powers) until the age of 61.

The quest for rejuvenation has also figured prominently from time to time in "scientific" experimentation, especially involving the sex glands. The French scientist Brown-Sequard believed that the secret of youthfulness, in men at least, lay in intravenous injections of animal testicles. Working along the same lines, a Viennese, Steinach, thought that tying off a man's spermatic cords would give him a sort of internal accumulation of sex hormones and make him young again. The Russian scientist, Voronov, went even further in his search for the elixir of youth. He transplanted monkey sex glands into both women and men. Metchnikoff, another Russian scientist, had an en-

8

tirely different theory. He believed that youth could be regained by ingesting special bacilli to "counteract" intestinal toxins which he thought were responsible for aging.

More recently, Dr. Saint-Pierre in France claims you are as old as your blood. He injects blood serum into older women and men in an effort to rejuvenate them.

There was much excitement in recent decades by reports that rejuvenation was possible by the injection of procaine (Novocaine), a local anesthetic. A Rumanian doctor, Ana Aslan, popularized this theory. She called her special preparation "H-3," alias Vitamin H-3, alias procaine. In 1951, she reported that the aging process could be retarded or reversed with procaine. In addition, she claimed miraculous benefit for a host of other conditions which commonly afflict the elderly—deafness, poor vision, impotence, heart disease, ulcers, hypertension, etc. She offered not a single controlled test or statistical analysis as evidence.

Nevertheless, the publicity her "treatments" received made scientists in this country and in England do their own research with procaine. They used the schedule Dr. Aslan recommended. The effects of procaine and those of a placebo (inactive) injection were exactly the same, except that sometimes hemorrhaging occurred with the procaine. The beneficial changes that did occur were probably a result of the elderly being particularly susceptible to suggestion. It is well known that patients receiving a new treatment— especially a "miraculous" one—will often feel better because they think they will.

Dr. Nathan Shock of the U.S. Institute of Health commented: "If these claims for procaine were true, you'd be adding 10 years to your life every time the dentist filled a tooth. This woman (Dr. Aslan) is the Pied Piper of the sixties, leading the aged instead of the young." And the American Medical Association's Council on Drugs urged physicians to disregard the therapeutic claims for procaine until and unless studies validate them.

In Switzerland, Dr. Paul Niehans has advocated the injection of cells of an unborn lamb into human beings to restore health and vitality. Dr. Niehans' treatment is not recognized in American medical circles, and the U.S. Food and Drug Administration forbids the importation of frozen or dried fetal animal cells into this country except for research purposes.

My own information about his methods comes from one of his disillusioned patients, who consulted me for menopausal symptoms.

This woman, now 56 years old, visited the Niehans Clinic about a year before she came to me. She had heard of revitalizing benefits of the doctor's "cellular therapy", and went to him because she had been feeling run-down. According to the document she had with her, she had been given "injections of fresh cells of: hypothalamus, placenta, marrow bone [sic], kidneys, thyroid, parathyroid, heart, arteries, ovaries, lobus frontalis, and adrenals". The cost was $1,300.

The following is the card she received on leaving the clinic:

To my patients!
Your organism has been given precious cells. I beg you not to damage them in any way! Therefore:
NO x-rays, no short-wave treatment, no ultraviolet rays,
NO bath-cures, in radio-active thermal stations,
NO sun baths, no Turkish baths, no sauna baths, no diathermy,
NO poisons, such as nicotine, concentrated alcohols, vaccines,
NO drugs (if possible) and no hormones.

Observe these instructions for the future, if you
wish the injected cells to be of help to you. Their
continued action depends entirely on you. These
instructions are for your whole life long.

Prof. Niehans

A few weeks after receiving the "cellular therapy", she
began getting hot flushes and sweats and had difficulty
sleeping (common menopausal symptoms of estrogen deficiency). She wrote to Dr. Niehans, and he told her that the
symptoms would disappear within three months. When
they didn't, she sought further medical help.

Her physical examination showed only vaginal atrophic
changes which indicated a considerable estrogen deficiency.
After a few weeks of estrogen medication, her symptoms
were gone and she felt well. In this case, treatment was
delayed unnecessarily while the patient waited for the effects
of a "revitalizer." The hormone pills she is now taking will
keep her from developing symptoms of estrogen deficiency.
But they will not make her any younger.

There are no rejuvenating pills. And the pill-takers
themselves seem to realize this. The story is told that Darryl
Zanuck and the Duke and Duchess of Windsor met Maurice
Chevalier at Maxim's in Paris. The Duke asked, "What kind
of pills does Chevalier take to look so young?" Zanuck
answered: "It's not that he takes pills. He doesn't. It's that
we do."

Chevalier isn't the only one who looks much younger
than his years. Whenever my secretary gives me the chart
of a new patient and there's a circle around her age, I know
that I may be surprised. A woman I'll call Mrs. G. gave her
age as 53. The very oldest she looked was 40. She had two
grown daughters—and three grandchildren. Her menopause was one year in the past, at which time she suffered
flushes and sweats for three months. She had had no
therapy at the time, and her symptoms had ceased spon-

11

taneously. Asked about her present complaints, she said she had none. But she had heard a lot about estrogen replacement therapy and said, "I'm not eager to take estrogen. I just want to know if I need it."

Physical examination disclosed no abnormalities. Her skin was remarkably young looking, with hardly a wrinkle. Her vaginal smears showed good estrogen activity. Of course, I told her no therapy was needed.

This woman picked her ancestors well. Her mother is 86 "but looks about 65." She has no sisters, but most of her mother's sisters died in their 90's "looking in their 60's." For her, youth was a gift.

Many other middle-aged women who *do* look their years ask about "pills to make me young again". Their wish for youth is really a wish to remain young-looking, which in our culture is a prerequisite for beauty. And pills to keep or make one beautiful do not exist.

Youth is not the *sine qua non* of beauty in all cultures. What one society considers beautiful another may not. We can't understand what a Zulu sees in his wife. And to satisfy some thirteenth century emperor's idea of beauty, the Chinese bound the feet of women until they were crippled. In Burma, the woman with the longest stretched neck is considered *la plus belle,* and the "duckbill" lipped Ubangi sends men into a tailspin. There's a waist-pinching tribe in New Guinea where the women look like an hourglass with not enough room for grains of sand to go through, let alone food.

But in our own culture, youth is the keynote. Youth means beauty. And in their quest, women go to beauty parlors, have their hair tinted, wear padded bras, don girdles, obtain contact lenses for their eyes and caps for their teeth, go on diets, use exercise machines, have nose bobs, and undergo face lifts.

Although attitudes toward aging vary from culture to culture, the wish to remain young or to regain youth has been universal throughout history. Women are particularly sensitive about growing older. It is hardly surprising that the current speculation about hormones to remain young, to postpone or even prevent the menopause and to slow the aging process has reawakened woman's dreams to be forever attractive, forever young.

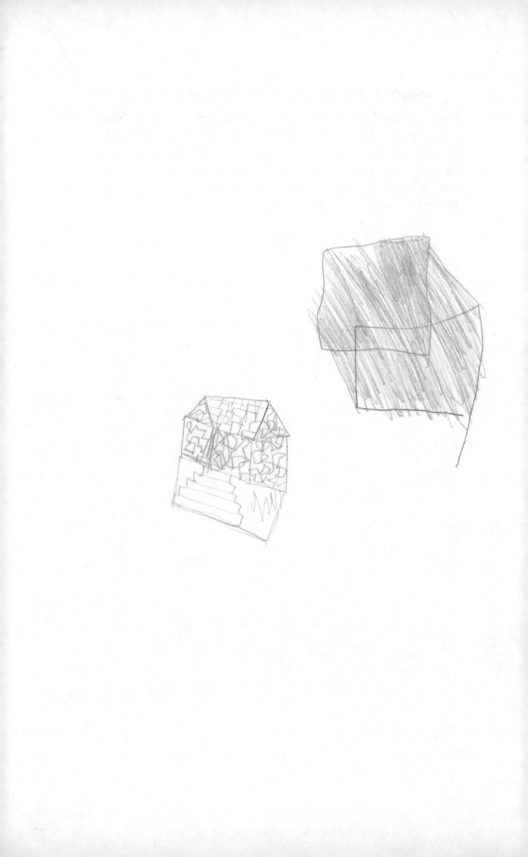

2

Change of Life . . . In a
Life of Change

Look abroad thro' Nature's range
Nature's mighty law is change
ROBERT BURNS

We must all grow older. Men do so gradually, without any major hormonal shifts. But women between the ages of 40 and 55 generally undergo a physiological change—the menopause. It's a curious coincidence that this age span constitutes a good chunk of what is known as middle age. For this period has its own share of problems. It seems that these two, menopause and middle age, are always being mistaken for each other. They shouldn't be.

The word "menopause" comes from the Greek words "month" and "cessation". It means a pause in the menses, or a cessation of monthly periods. The cause is a decrease of hormones produced by the ovaries. And the average age when this occurs is a little under 50. However, the age of menopause has been advancing steadily in recent decades in the United States and in most European countries, probably because of better health standards.

When a year has passed without menstruation, the menopause is considered fully established. This also marks the end of fertility.

The word "climacteric" also comes from two Greek words, one meaning "rung of a ladder" and the other "a critical time." That is, a step-by-step progression from

15

middle to old age, the process being "critical". Climacteric is a more comprehensive term than menopause, and refers to a *span* of time during which the menopause occurs. The climacteric age range is roughly from 40 to 60. This is also middle age!

The popular term "Change of Life" is used to indicate either menopause or climacteric. It implies the departure of a former life and the emergence of a new one. But the new one connotes regression or degeneration—that is, toward an advanced age.

The expression "going through the change" has even more ominous overtones, like steering a dangerous course through choppy waters. In fact, those women who are fortunate enough not to have any particular discomforts at this time are often described as having "sailed through" the menopause.

For all women the menopause is but one climacteric change in a life of changes. There's the sweeping hormonal and personality change from girlhood to womanhood, the extraordinary hormonal changes during pregnancy, and finally the hormonal shift called menopause. How a woman reacts emotionally to menopausal changes usually is similar to how she has reacted to the other changes.

In our culture, the transition from little girl to adolescent requires a marked shift in social behavior and personality. In other cultures, where childhood conditioning prepares a girl explicitly and continuously for her female role, the transition from childhood to adolescence is rarely traumatic.

Writing about our society, Margaret Mead has said, "Women's lives are arranged in sharp, discontinuous steps, with the emphasis almost inevitably on being a virgin, a girl who has ceased to be a virgin, a childless woman, a woman who has borne a child, a woman [past menopause] who can no longer bear a child."

16

In cultures where the onset of menstruation is taken most casually, so is its cessation. But in societies where the little girl is sharply differentiated from the potentially fertile young woman, so is the woman past menopause—the infertile woman—distinguished from her younger sisters. Under such circumstances, one can understand how the menopause may produce anxiety, and how this may be followed by a denial of the change—with resulting depression.

Many women today await menopause with a dread more appropriate to a descent into Dante's Inferno. Many expect signs that are equally dreadful—ranging from cancer to insanity. Such wisdom, no doubt, can be supported by old wives' tales and family lore—"Grandmother died of cancer . . . she was in her change, you know." Or, "Poor Aunt Clara . . . going through the menopause and ending in an asylum like that. . . ."

In this we are neither alone nor unique. Of course, past cultures didn't have much of a menopause problem, since most people didn't live that long. Yet history does yield evidence that the postmenopausal woman saw herself—and was seen by her society—in a significantly changed role.

In some cultures, taboos were lifted with the onset of the menopause. They believed that the "change of life" (which was equated with a long life) conferred protective virtues on a woman. For example, only postmenopausal Ashanti women were permitted near sacred shrines. In various tribes, women of this age group were also given greater freedom in conversation and were excused from unpleasant tasks. Sometimes the menopausal honors turned out to be rather dubious. For instance, a Creek warrior wounded in battle could be attended only by a woman "past the age of sinning with men".

In societies that did not completely ban exposure of the female genitals, it was the young girl—and the woman

17

past menopause—who was allowed to go naked. In these societies, menopause was truly a *"retour d'age,"* a return to young age as the French call it.

A book on menopause written about seventy years ago shows that human nature hasn't changed much.

> Races and nations which are phlegmatic, cold, and apathetic, women who are inured to out-of-door life and severe manual labor, savage and barbarous women, peasants, Germans, Scandinavians, and Russians, are apt to complain little of the experiences of the menopause; while the sensitive, passionate nations like the French, Spanish and Irish, the highly organized, nervous, city-bred women, women of fashion, women who fret and worry, are apt to experience the disagreeable and annoying features of the menopause.

There's evidence that menopause was a problem in the United States even in the nineteenth century. (At the turn of the century the average life span for women was only 49 years.) It is interesting to read the medical writings of that time, when knowledge of physiology was meager and female hormones were still undiscovered. An 1894 article from the *Journal of the American Medical Association* pinpointed the cardinal symptoms of the menopause:

> The symptoms of the menopause are: a. cessation of the monthly flow; b. flashes of heat; c. flushes of circulation; d. irregular perspiration. . . .

But the doctor was on less sure ground when it came to guessing the cause:

> The first thing I search for in such a woman is diseased genitals, e.g., endometritis [infection] is the arch fiend.

The author also believed menopause was due to atrophy of the uterus rather than the ovaries.

As for the treatment of the day, certain specific measures were recommended: ". . . hot douches gradually increased up to ten quarts twice daily." For insomnia: "The bromids act well." Regarding bowels: "The bowels are best regulated by having the patient drink a glass of water each night at bedtime in which there is from half to a drachm of Epsom salts. . . ." As for sex: "Excessive sexual desire at the menopause is indicative of disease." And then:

> Such patients have so much lack of confidence in themselves, their physicians and their friends that they have not the will power to keep up a systemic course of treatment. Hence they go around from one physician to another.

Less than forty years later, when more was known about hormonal physiology, some medical writers strongly condemned indifference toward the menopause. For example, note how the following excerpt from a 1932 medical journal resembles some highly publicized present-day writings of those who have taken up the cudgel for hormonal therapy:

> The immediate and various symptoms which women show at this time are often disregarded by the physician, and the only answer often given the patient is that she should not worry about her condition as it is an unavoidable consequence of her age and will subside in a short time without treatment. This attitude is absolutely wrong because it gives poor service to the patient, and the physician omits many opportunities for satisfactory treatment, since most of the symptoms

can be alleviated by proper advice once they are recognized as being due to the climacterium.

This was written at a time when hormonal therapy was not yet in general use. But the writer knew that the menopause could be associated with many disagreeable symptoms, uniquely female.

It seems to me that anthropologists have given us valuable data from which much practical information can be drawn. The knowledge that reaction to a physiological process such as menstruation or menopause can be culturally influenced is important. It would seem, therefore, that a woman's "preparation" for menopause must start in childhood. As with so many other "changes," her psychological adaptation to the menopause will depend largely on the way she accepts her changing role. Hormone therapy has solved some of the physical and physiological problems related to menopause. But there are other problems at this time of life that refuse to disappear with the taking of pills. They are problems of middle age.

When does middle age begin? Is it "when you are too young to take up golf and too old to rush up to the net?" Men seem to thrive on middle age. Income is usually highest at this time; professional advancement at its peak. Many prominent people in our government are men in their forties and fifties. As far as physical fitness goes, several of our astronauts are over forty. Middle agers occupy the seats of power and foot the bills. They are "The Command Generation."

But how does woman accept middle age? Not with open arms, but with clenched fists. There are just too many "changes" going on at this time—changes which threaten her womanhood. She is concerned with each added year, each added pound, each new gray hair. She worries that she is becoming less attractive to her husband. If he is busier than ever and seems less attentive, she interprets this as rejection. Her children may have grown to the point of no longer "needing" her. She may find it difficult to keep a job, or get a new one. If she is single, she sees her chances of marriage slipping away with each passing year. If, on the other hand, she had been happily married and is now widowed, she must adjust to an irreplaceable loss.

In short, she sees loneliness ahead. This is the time of life when regrets and recriminatons begin to creep in—"If only I had done this . . . If only I had done that. . . ." She begins taking a sleeping pill at night, and tranquilizers during the day. Perhaps a couple of extra drinks now and then. She may become moody and depressed, suffer from fatigue, backache, insomnia, headaches.

And it is in this setting that menopause arrives. It couldn't come at a worse time.

Menopause can bring its own discomforts and problems. Some are strikingly similar to the problems and symptoms of middle age—depression and fatigue, irritability, insomnia. Since menopause occurs during middle age it is often difficult to decide which symptoms are attributable to which cause. But we do know that even mild menopausal symptoms, *if superimposed on nonmenopausal symptoms,* can be overburdening. The treatment of one must necessarily be related to the other. They cannot be separated. Thus, to the burdens of menopause with its hormonal changes are added the anxieties and stresses of middle age. It is hard enough to cope with one. But when you have to take a double dose at a crucial period in life, it can be a heavy burden.

Can hormones help? They cannot solve emotional problems. But they can prevent or relieve the physical symptoms of menopause. And this makes a woman better able to face the psychological problems of middle aging.

Not all middle-aged women go into a tailspin. Many suffer no menopausal discomforts. They are fortunate. This isn't entirely chance. Menopausal symptoms have two components, physical and emotional. If there is little or no discomfort, the woman is probably physically and emotionally healthy. There are many such women. Physiologically they maintain an adequate though not necessarily high estrogen level. And they suffer no deficiency symptoms.

The psychologically healthy middle-aged woman does not fall prey to the youth cult. She does not lament bygone years. If she reflects on the past, she reflects on her successes—not her failures. She finds pleasure in her family, her friends, her pursuits. She enjoys life.

3

Hormones, Sex Glands,
and Menopause

Woman's at best a contradiction still!
ALEXANDER POPE

Nature has seen to our reproduction.

The testicles or testes of a man correspond to the ovaries in a woman. The testes produce sperm—about one quarter billion per ejaculation. The ovaries, which start out with about a half million unripe eggs in childhood, release one a month for some thirty years—about four hundred eggs altogether.

It doesn't seem possible that only three hundred years ago sperm were completely unknown. The first one to see them was Johann Ham, a pupil of Leeuwenhoek, inventor of the microscope.

Upon discovery of sperm, two opposing schools sprang up. One group insisted that sperm originated life; the other, that the egg was responsible. Amazingly, for the next hundred years no one thought of the answer—that it required the marriage of the two!

Let's consider woman's biological role in this process.

Let's consider her endocrine or glandular system. Not the glands of *external* secretion, which produce visible products such as saliva or tears. But rather the glands of *internal* secretion, the ductless glands that pour out their powerful hormones directly into the blood stream. The main ductless glands are the pituitary, ovaries, thyroid and adrenals.

23

The glandular system is often compared to an orchestra. The "master gland"—the pituitary—is the conductor. It directs the other glands and makes them play louder or softer according to the body's requirements. By a delicate feedback mechanism, the pituitary is also influenced by the same glands it affects.

However, the pituitary actually is more a figurehead than a master gland. It takes orders, behind the scenes of course, from a powerful impresario called the hypothalamus (midbrain).

According to latest theory, nerve endings in a portion of the hypothalamus release "neurohumors". These are carried to the anterior pituitary, where they control hormonal output.

In experiments with animals, the pituitary was transplanted from the base of the skull to muscle tissues of the body, at which time menstrual function ceased. When it was transplanted back to its original position, menstrual function resumed. Apparently, it needed this contact with the hypothalamus. Thus, the pituitary is really the hypothalamus' servant.

The hypothalamus is about as big as a walnut, and it forms the walls of the third brain ventricle. It is often called the seat of human feeling and emotion. Basically it is a coordinating center, a sort of neural switchboard through which myriad impulses pass in a way infinitely more intricate than any man-made computer. Emotions can affect the hypothalamus and thus indirectly affect the pituitary. This helps explain how emotions can influence physiological functions. An obvious example is the young woman who misses one or two menstrual periods because she *fears* she is pregnant.

So complex is the glandular system that one literally cannot tell the players without a program. Some definitions, therefore, are in order.

Whenever most people think of hormones, they usually do so in association with the sex glands. The word "hormone" is derived from the Greek. It means "to arouse or set in motion." Hormones are secreted by the endocrine glands. But there is evidence that some are produced also by cells without recognizable glandular structure.

Most of us tend to take hormones for granted, and forget how powerful they are. Only when an obvious or dramatic irregularity occurs do we take notice. For example, if the pancreas does not secrete enough insulin hormone the result is diabetes. When the thyroid is markedly deficient from birth, a cretin develops. Perhaps the most startling example of a gland gone berserk is gigantism or dwarfism, as seen in circus sideshows.

The sex hormones (or sex steroids, as they are sometimes called) include estrogen and progesterone in the woman, and androgen (testosterone) in the man. They are all in the steroid family, much like first cousins. Estrogen and progesterone are produced mainly in the ovaries of the nonpregnant woman. Testosterone is produced mainly in the testes of the man. However, women also produce small quantities of male hormone, and men produce some estrogen, but not progesterone. (Ovaries and testes are also called "gonads", from the Greek *"gone"* which means "seed.")

The adrenal hormones (or adrenal steroids) are produced by two adrenal glands which are situated one on top of each kidney. The best known adrenal hormone is "adrenaline," always called for in "Dr. Kildare-type dramas" to revive a failing heart. More familiarly it is responsible for the rapid beating of the heart during flight or fright. The outer cover of the adrenal produces many cortisone-type hormones which have been modified to treat various arthritic, inflammatory and allergic conditions.

About three hundred years ago, a Dutch physician named De Graaf first linked the ovaries to reproduction. He suggested the name "ovary" because he assumed, incorrectly, that an ovarian follicle corresponded to a bird's nest.

The human egg follicle which matures each month of reproductive life is known as the Graafian follicle.

It was not until 1923 that estrogen, the chief "female" hormone of the ovary, was isolated from follicular fluid by Allen and Doisy. Estrogen is really a collective word meaning "estrogenic hormones." There are three main ones—estradiol, which is the most potent, is readily transformed in the body to estrone, which in turn can be changed to estriol. Estrogen makes a girl a woman. It is responsible for the growth and development of her breasts, genitals, axillary and pubic hair, and body contours. With the other ovarian hormone, progesterone, it shares responsibility for the menstrual cycle. In fact, estrogen dominates the cycle at the time of puberty and again as menopause approaches.

The primary source of estrogen is the ovaries. But during pregnancy it's manufactured in huge quantities by the placenta. One of the best sources of "natural" estrogen is the pregnant mare, which excretes in the urine more than 100 mg daily. (Surprisingly, the stallion secretes even more. In fact, the virile stallion puts more estrogen into its environment than any other living creature.)

There is evidence that estrogen is also produced by the adrenal glands, and that this is an important source of estrogen for the postmenopausal woman. There are probably other sources. In an unusual experimental study of breast cancer cases where ovaries, adrenals and pituitary were all removed, measurable levels of estrogen were still found in the urine. Where did it come from? No one knows for sure.

There is little estrogen in common foods. However, there apparently was enough estrogen in Australian clover to act as a birth control pill, causing sterility in grazing sheep.

In a normal cycle, a woman produces only about 5 mg of estrogen. By contrast, during the latter part of her pregnancy she may produce about 600 times that amount.

When a woman becomes pregnant, the embryonic tissue secretes a hormone, chorionic gonadotropin, about a week after implantation. This is responsible for the "positive" pregnancy test. At around the third month, the developing placenta begins to secrete progesterone in earnest, as well as estrogen, enough so that the ovaries are no longer needed.

With all of the steps and chemical interchanges that must take place for a single normal menstrual cycle, it's a wonder that things don't go haywire more often. Every single player in the orchestra must play in harmony. One sour note and the conductor will wave his baton furiously.

The menstrual cycle depends upon smooth hormonal interaction. The first half of the cycle is dominated by estrogen, produced by maturing follicles (egg sacs) in the ovaries. The ovaries are spurred on by the pituitary gonadotropic hormones. Specifically, the follicle-stimulating hormone (FSH) of the pituitary causes one of the follicles to mature, usually once a month. About two weeks before menstruation, this follicle ruptures and extrudes an egg. Now, under the influence of another pituitary gonadotropic hormone, the "luteinizing hormone" (LH), the remaining egg sac is transformed into a "corpus luteum" (yellow body). This now secretes both estrogen and progesterone to prepare the lining of the womb for a possible pregnancy. If there is no fertilization, the corpus luteum stops functioning and its hormones are sharply withdrawn, resulting in the shedding of the uterine lining. This is menstruation.

If pregnancy *does* take place, the shell from which the ovum was extruded continues to function, producing much more estrogen and progesterone. A few weeks later, the placenta takes over the function of producing these hormones, and continues to do so right up to the time of delivery.

Thus the ovaries and pituitary are the chief glands

concerned with menstruation and reproduction. And the hypothalamus always lurks in the background. For smooth functioning, however, it's also important for two other glands—the thyroid and the adrenals—to cooperate. They too influence menstruation, fertility, and the menopause.

The reason few women experience extremely severe menopausal symptoms is that ovarian hormonal function generally does not stop abruptly. It does so gradually. Only if the ovaries are removed do symptoms usually become sudden and severe.

What happens when the ovaries begin to fail in middle age? There is a decreased production of estrogen and an increased production of pituitary follicle-stimulating hormone. This is the result of the pituitary's effort to stimulate an unresponsive ovary. And there is no progesterone production by the postmenopausal ovaries, since that stopped months before, when ovulation ceased.

But the ovaries still put out a measurable amount of estrogen. This estrogen production declines gradually to a plateau. But by then the main source of estrogen is probably the adrenal glands. Removal of the ovaries may not reduce the estrogen level below a certain point, but removal of the adrenals does. Also, the high pituitary secretion, if undisturbed, is maintained for many years, decreasing only after the age of sixty or seventy, possibly as a result of natural aging.

Thyroid function in normal postmenopausal women seems to change very little. Perhaps there's a slight decrease with the years. The adrenal glands after menopause probably continue to secrete not only estrogen but also some progesterone.

With the decline of the sex hormones—estrogen and progesterone—we see gradual evidence of the physiological changes that take place in a woman.

Although other mammals are able to reproduce till their last years, the human female can't. Her reproductive

28

function ends when menopause is established; because the ovaries, which used to release an egg each month for possible fertilization, cease doing so once menstruation has permanently stopped. Apparently this is due to the natural aging of human ovaries and cannot be altered by any known means, hormonal or otherwise. That is, even if menstrual periods are restored by regular hormone taking, the result is only artificial bleeding. No egg is passed. There is no fertility.

Along with the absence of the reproductive function there is an abrupt decline in progesterone production. No egg, no progesterone. However, estrogen production declines much more gradually. The ovaries can manufacture estrogen even without egg formation. Lower levels of estrogen are measurable from the fiftieth year on. Apparently even the aged, so-called atrophic ovary can still manufacture some estrogen, as seen when postmenopausal women whose ovaries are ultimately removed suddenly develop menopausal symptoms.

Exactly how estrogen alleviates typical menopausal symptoms such as flushes and sweating is still not known. Some feel that estrogen helps by causing a release of pituitary luteinizing hormone, but others have found a natural increase in this hormone with or without symptoms or therapy. Most researchers agree, though, that flushes are related to dilatation of tiny arteries. At the same time, almost all observers have noted the relationship of flushes to aggravation from psychological, social or medical problems. In this respect, all roads again seem to lead to the hypothalamus, and involve the heat-regulating center.

Physiologic changes occur as a woman grows older, but the exact role of estrogen lack in many of the changes is not clear. Obviously the greatest effects of diminished estrogen production will be on those *target* organs which, in their development, had the most to do with ovarian sex hormones—the breasts and genital organs.

The breasts at first have a tendency to become fatty during middle age. But, with advancing years, the fat is absorbed and they become smaller and flabbier. The uterus gradually gets smaller. The lining of the uterus may at first show a thickening due to estrogen stimulation unopposed by progesterone, but gradually it too becomes thin and atrophic. The cervical canal leading to the uterus becomes very narrow.

The lining of the vagina is sensitive to hormonal fluctuations and may show early signs of estrogen deprivation by gradually losing its elastic tissue and becoming thin, sometimes to the point of tiny ulcerations. The urethra (opening leading to the bladder) and part of the bladder itself undergo a similar process of thinning.

There is also loss of fatty tissue from the external vaginal lips, which gradually become smaller, as do the internal lips. The vaginal walls may become relaxed from loss of muscle tone.

There is a tendency—nonhormonal—to gain weight, with a redistribution of fat during middle age. After about age 65, weight tends to remain at a plateau until about 80, when it begins to decrease. You seldom see fat women of 80.

There is also a gradual loss of kidney function with advancing age due to decreased blood flow through the kidneys. Systolic blood pressure increases rather gradually until about the age of 65 before leveling off.

Decreased strength, speed and endurance are also the result of aging, as any middle-aged parent who has ever raced with his adolescent children can testify. The healing of bone and tissue is also slower with advancing years, hence the great fear of fractures in the elderly.

Other more subtle changes that occur with age include decreased tissue elasticity, cellular degeneration, atrophy of nerve tissue and increased pigmentation. Skin tone is diminished. There is also a shrinking of the total mass of organs, perhaps as a result of loss of intracellular water, nitrogen, phosphorus and potassium.

Mental changes are probably produced by a general atrophy of the brain. It is common to have a loss of memory, especially for recent events.

The effect of estrogen on the physiological changes mentioned is variable. For instance, in the case of a target organ such as the uterus, if one gives even an 80-year-old woman enough ovarian hormones, her uterus can be stimulated to respond even to the point of menstruation. Vaginal atrophy also responds well to estrogen as do urethral atrophic changes. Other changes, however, are not that specific. And there's no evidence at all that hormone therapy will increase your total life span. All body cells and systems are involved in the aging process. Only some of them are related to the endocrine glands and their hormonal secretions. To our frustration, the cause of aging remains unknown.

૭

4

How You Feel

*Better a blush on the cheek
than a spot on the heart*
CERVANTES

❧

How many physical symptoms arising during middle age
are caused by a hormone deficiency?

The answer ranges from few to many, depending upon
which medical article you read. One report, for example,
lists 11 specific menopausal symptoms. Another lists no less
than 28. I recently reviewed the histories of two hundred
menopausal or postmenopausal patients in my practice,
each of whom related her own complaints to menopause
according to what she had heard or read in various publica-
tions. There were almost 50 different symptoms!

This is only one of the many controversial aspects of
menopause. Let's see if the knot can be untangled.

There's a common denominator among the many
complaints, aside from cessation of the menstrual periods.
The cardinal symptoms are hot flushes and sweating. To
these may be added vaginal discomfort due to a thinning of
the vaginal lining. Emotional states and changes in appearance are sometimes referred to as "associated" or "secondary" menopausal complaints.

How many women complain about menopausal symptoms? One survey of women *who sought medical help*
found that only 10 percent were severely affected by menopausal symptoms. Another writer said that only about 15
percent of menopausal women require therapy, another

33

about 30 percent. From my own experience, I'd say that the incidence of complaints of those seeking medical help, *traceable in whole or part to the hormonal shift of the menopause,* is closer to 50 percent.

But percentages mean little to the individual woman who is troubled. She wants relief. She requires attention regardless of the origin of her complaints. Besides, the clinical symptoms of distress vary greatly, even in the same individual, due to differing physical and emotional demands that aggravate the symptoms. And, happily, many postmenopausal women have no symptoms at all. They apparently continue to produce enough estrogen for many years.

Hot flushes and sweats are typical menopausal symptoms. But high blood pressure can also produce heat feelings similar to menopausal flushes, and sweating is common in anxiety states or with an overactive thyroid. In general, however, flushes and sweats are symptomatic of the menopause.

The terms "flushes" and "flashes" are used interchangeably. You could say that waves of heat involving the head and upper body may appear so suddenly as to be called flashes, and the reddening of the skin or blushing that often accompanies that feeling is called flushes. The sensation lasts about as long as a labor pain, thirty to forty seconds. It is often followed by sweating. The symptoms can be most distressing, particularly at night, resulting in insomnia, irritability and nervousness.

Surprisingly, the exact cause of menopausal flushes and sweats remains unknown! But it's generally conceded that these symptoms are among the few which do have a genuine hormonal basis. Some observers have thought that increased pituitary secretion is to blame. Most clinicians agree that decreased estrogen production plays a role since it has been found that estrogen relieves the symptoms, even in dosages that do not alter the level of pituitary secretions. Yet there are missing pieces to the puzzle. Neither of these theories satisfactorily explains why flushes are only temporary and subside spontaneously in the untreated woman, even though the hormonal changes persist. Also unexplained is why some women, despite diminished estrogen production, never have flushes and others have the symptom for years. Also, flushes which have long disappeared can suddenly reappear years later when the woman is under stress. So a deficiency in estrogen cannot explain *all* cases. Severe estrogen lack in *young* women with ovarian failure is usually *not* associated with flushes. It does seem to follow that a woman must have had years of exposure to estrogen for the hypothalamus to react with "heated displeasure" upon the withdrawal of hormonal support.

Whatever the cause, it's obvious that something is affecting a woman's heat-regulating mechanism to produce these annoying vasomotor symptoms. Flushes are aggravated by anything which diminishes heat loss or stimulates heat production—exercise, eating, heavy bedclothes, warm weather, stress. The degree and severity of vasomotor symptoms varies in different women. Some individuals never experience a single flush; others have mild, transient symptoms. Others have drenching sweats and flushes visible to the observer. Whatever the degree, flushes are almost always annoying. I say almost because, when I started to tell one woman that her flushes could be helped, she interrupted and said, "I should say *not*. They come in very handy in the cold weather!"

Although flushes are most common after menstrual periods have ceased, they may occur while a woman is still having periods, though other "changes" such as scanty flow or wider spacing between periods will usually be noted. The unusual woman who complains of flushes while having regular menstrual periods is not in the "menopause". An understanding of her hormonal status may be obtained by vaginal smears, by measuring her pituitary hormonal gonadotropic secretions, or by a therapeutic test with estrogen. The latter, at the same time, relieves symptoms due to any estrogen deficiency.

Although flushes have been helped by sedatives, tranquilizers, placebos and plain talk, the most effective treatment is with estrogen. Relief is dramatic.

It wasn't always so. In previous generations, those women who lived long enough to have menopausal vasomotor symptoms could look forward to no specific remedy. Hormones were unknown. A good description of how little could be done for them is found in the following excerpt from a medical book on the menopause published in 1897:

> [For] vasomotor troubles, blushes, flashes of heat with possible subsequent profuse perspiration . . . which sometimes persists until advanced life . . . such women should always pay close attention to the condition of the gastrointestinal canal, their diet should be simple and wholesome; alcohol, spices, highly seasoned food should be abstained from; the bowels should be kept freely open . . . encourage free elimination through the skin by exercise, friction, and frequent bathing in water at a temperature of 60° to 70° F.
>
> [For] the congestions of the genital organs, which are sometimes particularly distressing in causing sexual excitement . . . relief may often be obtained by the abstraction of blood from the *os uteri* either with leeches or by means of puncture with a tenaculum or scalpel, an ounce or more of blood being removed. [For] sweating, atropine sulphate has been recommended. . . .
>
> There is little additional which can be said

in regard to the general treatment of those who are passing through the menopause. Those who are not sick, but think they are, must be disillusioned with gentleness but firmness.

So one is fortunate to be living in the present. Leeches are hard to get.

Flushes, along with bloodletting, should be a thing of the past. Sometimes a woman will report that sweating is even more troublesome than the flushes. Typical comments: "Water runs from me like a faucet"; "I'm bathed in perspiration every night"; "Drenched." Sweating, as I have mentioned, need not necessarily be due to menopause. It can be triggered by excitement or anxiety—for example, the "wet paw syndrome". Other conditions associated with troublesome sweating are thyroid excess and tuberculosis. Some people perspire a lot after taking alcohol or aspirin, others just from eating spicy or hot foods.

Among my patients troubled with prolonged flushes and mild sweating was a woman I'll call Mrs. S. She was a tall, heavy-set woman of 58, extroverted, with no unusual emotional problems. Her home and family seemed to provide her with basic satisfactions. She had experienced the menopause eight years before I saw her, and had suffered no complaints except for flushes and sweats which, after eight years, still showed no signs of abating. The physical examination was normal, except for showing a slight estrogen deficiency on the smear. A small dose of estrogen quickly relieved the flushes. The dose schedule was later modified to once every three days. It she stops taking the estrogen for more than two or three weeks, the flushes return. On one occasion, a mild sedative was substituted for the estrogen. The flushes returned, so she is back on a small dose of estrogen and feels fine.

It is not uncommon for an emotional situation to precipitate the onset of menopausal or postmenopausal flushes. Another one of my patients, Mrs. N., had at 54 experienced her last period two years previously. She had been doing well, without any complaints, until the previous month, when the marriage of her only daughter seemed to be breaking up. At that point her flushes returned, and were relieved by a small dose of estrogen. Since then Mrs. N. has been taking estrogen cyclically. It seems to help her cope more successfully with her problems. (Her daughter, incidentally, was recently divorced. And the shock wasn't as great as Mrs. N. feared it would be.)

Some women experience flushes periodically, every few months or even every few years—usually coincidental with some upheaval or anxiety in their lives. Does the estrogen level happen to drop at such periods? I think not. More likely, the heat-regulating centers become disturbed by the emotional turmoil.

In some patients, large doses of estrogen are required to relieve estrogen-related symptoms and create a sense of well-being. This was true of Mrs. B. At 49, she was happily married, though childless, and she had had the menopause three years before. Flushes, sweats, vaginal discomfort, insomnia, fatigue,—she had them all! Yet her physical examination showed nothing wrong except for marked thinning of the vaginal tissues. Although oral and local estrogen therapy were begun, it was soon noted that, according to her symptoms and vaginal smear response, the average dose of estrogen caused only slight improvement. By regulating the dosage according to the effect on her symptoms, I found that she needed three or four times the usual dose to maintain a state of well-being. On a high dosage, all her symptoms disappeared. "This has given me a new lease on life," she said.

A very common middle age affliction is backache. And in postmenopausal women, backache is sometimes associated with osteoporosis, a thinning of the bone. Osteoporosis is somehow related to estrogen. But backache, it should be noted, is a symptom, not a diagnosis. Its causes are many, and osteoporosis is only one of them.

Hardly anyone—man or woman—reaches middle age without experiencing some sort of back trouble. It often follows a strain, such as improper lifting without bending the knees. In the ordinary aging process, muscles and tendons begin to lose some of their elasticity. Putting on weight, sleeping on a soft mattress, standing for long periods and poor posture all contribute to backache. Inactivity is another common cause. Many a stiff back has been cured by a brisk walk each day.

So the most common cause of backache is lumbosacral or other ligamentous strain. Another fairly common cause, surprisingly, is intense emotional strain.

Arthritis is another middle age troublemaker. Of the various arthritic disorders, a few dominate. Joint problems may come from an injury, an infection, or metabolic and nutritive disorders. So-called "arthritic joint pain" is a loose term. It refers to the vague pains of middle- and older-age groups, and afflicts women more often than men. There is no evidence linking such disorders to hormone deficiency, and there is no logical explanation why these pains are sometimes relieved by estrogens. But they may be even though no improvement can be seen on x-ray.

Mrs. Y. came to me with the complaint of osteoporosis (bone thinning). This had been diagnosed by x-rays. She was 57, married and the mother of three grown children. For the previous eighteen months, she had been on calcium therapy and had exercised religiously. The improvement was moderate, but there was still enough discomfort to make her unhappy. She did have a moderate degree of osteoporosis of the spine, and signs of moderate estrogen deficiency.

I prescribed estrogen. Her remaining discomfort, particularly the back pain, disappeared. Once again she was able to resume the physical work which she enjoyed. It isn't at all clear why estrogen should give symptomatic relief of osteoporosis. But it does. And it has done as much for women in similar situations, as many orthopedists can testify. Estrogen therapy seems to prevent further progress of the disorder, at least for the time being.

Osteoarthritis has nothing to do with osteoporosis. With the former, there's characteristically an ache in the joint, worse on motion and relieved by rest. Yet, after rest, there is usually an increased stiffness, with pain gradually easing on motion. Apparently wear and tear increases the severity of this form of rheumatism. This is why it's more common in manual laborers than in those with sedentary occupations. There is a gradual wearing away of the cartilage and membrane surrounding the joints, causing bone to rub against bone, with resulting pain. Changes in the weather are thought to aggravate this condition. Aspirin and various other drugs are employed in symptomatic treatment. Estrogens appear to play no role. Moving to a different climate sometimes helps. But, oddly enough, a warm climate is better for some sufferers, a cold one better for others. Some patients with advanced osteoarthritis have very few complaints. Others with minor cases have considerable discomfort.

As for "spa" therapy, an article in the *Journal of the American Medical Association* attributed the benefits to "rest, relaxation, freedom from responsibility, change of environment, and possible diet, rather than . . . the baths themselves."

"Housemaid's knee" or "tennis elbow" is caused by inflammation of a bursa or joint capsule, as are "golfer's wrist," "pitcher's arm" and other inflamed joints. Estrogen plays no role here. Treatment is with heat, aspirin or injections of hydrocortisone directly into the inflamed area.

Three times as many women as men suffer from rheumatoid arthritis. The cause of this is unknown, as is the cure. Here too, aspirin, cortisone-type drugs, gold salts and other drugs are used. Physiotherapy is important. Estrogen seems to be completely unrelated.

෪

5

Hormones and Cancer

Fear may be . . . due to a mental picture of some destructive or painful evil in the future
ARISTOTLE

ꙮ

"But doctor, I've heard that hormones can cause cancer," said the woman in my consultation room, puffing deeply on her cigarette.

If my mind seemed far away at the moment, it was. I was thinking of an ad run by the American Cancer Society: "Last year, 300,000 Americans finally quit smoking." This line appeared beneath a picture of a graveyard.

It is strange that people will cling to myth and un-proved fears, and at the same time ignore opportunities for cancer prevention where the evidence of hazard to health *is* overwhelming. I have lost count of the number of women who have sat across my desk, chain-smoking, and at the same time expressing their fear of cancer from taking hormones. Yet in the minds of many, the word "hormone" is almost synonymous with cancer.

How did this fear get started?

It began perhaps back in 1932 with experiments on hereditary breast cancer in mice. A French scientist showed that spaying early in life prevented the development of cancer in female mice and, conversely, breast cancer was produced in *male* mice belonging to a cancer-susceptible strain by administering huge amounts of estrogen to

43

them over a long period of time. But he was unable to produce such cancer in mice belonging to a strain in which spontaneous breast cancer seldom occurred in the females. Similar experiments some years later have shown that cancer can develop in estrogen-fed offspring of mice, but only if the mothers belong to a cancer-susceptible strain. A woman would have to swallow about 150 pounds of estrogen over half her lifetime to receive a dose comparable to that in the mouse experiments.

So much for mice. How about other animals? Dogs and rabbits never develop mammary cancer as a result of estrogen administration. Similar experiments have been carried out in monkeys, which bear a much closer resemblance to humans both physiologically and organically. Injecting monkeys with large doses of estrogens has consistently failed to show any harmful effects, even when such injections were given for prolonged periods of time.

What about cancer of the *uterus* in animal experiments? Such work has been done, and it was not possible to produce uterine cancer in monkeys even by long-term estrogen stimulation. In fact, it has been practically impossible to induce cancer in the lining of the womb with estrogens in any experimental animals.

The particular susceptibility of certain strains of animals to certain disorders, or to a particular reaction, is known as "species specificity". It does not necessarily follow that such reactions can be applied to humans. For example, if you feed meat to a canary it may die. But this hardly means that meat is lethal for humans.

Cancer of the breast and reproductive tract in women seems to occur more often when there is *less* estrogen in the body, rather than more. For example, over 90 percent of cancers of the uterus occur in women past forty years of age, a time when their estrogen stores are diminishing. The incidence of breast cancer also increases with age.

During pregnancy, a woman's ovaries pour out enormous quantities of estrogen into her blood stream. Yet the incidence of breast malignancy is no greater among pregnant women than in the nonpregnant. In fact, less. Even with women who have had many children in rapid succession, hence an almost continuous high concentration of estrogen, cancer during pregnancy remains relatively rare.

Finally, the incidence and the mortality rate of breast cancer is just about the same today as it was back in 1930, when estrogens were not in general use. Literally tons of estrogen have been prescribed by doctors since that time for many purposes, including estrogens contained in contraceptive pills. All of this has made no appreciable difference in the statistics, showing no increase in deaths from cancer of the breast or uterus. This fact, perhaps more than any other, refutes the fear that estrogens cause cancer.

Nevertheless, let's take a look at all sides of the picture. After all, if there is *any* concern by reputable physicians or scientists that hormonal administration may cause cancer, this concern is for the patient's welfare.

The concern that cancer of the uterine lining and estrogen are somehow related stems from statistical data. When estrogen alone is given over a prolonged time, especially if uninterrupted, there is a tendency for the uterine lining to pile up (hyperplasia). Uterine cancer may coexist with or follow hyperplasia, particularly a less common but more active form called adenomatous (tumor-like) hyperplasia. But it is unjustified to conclude that estrogen actually causes the cancer. Some medical investigators have disagreed with the hyperplasia-cancer tie-up. The statistics have also been questioned. And the over-all evidence implicating estrogen is meager.

The tendency of estrogen administration to cause uterine hyperplasia can usually be minimized by cyclic therapy in the lowest effective dosage, or by adding progesterone. Progesterone is the natural antagonist of estrogen, and it has been demonstrated in both animals and humans that uterine hyperplasia can undergo regression when progesterone is given. This quality of progesterone has been increasingly used therapeutically, not only in cases of uterine hyperplasia but even in some cases of uterine cancer, with promising beneficial effects.

Some observers have reported an increased incidence of uterine cancer associated with estrogen-producing tumors of the ovary, and also in certain glandular imbalances which permit the body's own estrogen to act in a prolonged, unopposed manner, including women with late menopause. These statistics, too, have been challenged.

Working backwards, so to speak, there have been a few relatively small surveys of the incidence of uterine (and breast) malignancies during prolonged estrogen therapy. Most have reported no cases of cancer at all. However, it has been correctly pointed out that it really requires much broader studies involving much larger numbers of women and carefully documented data over a great many years, to arrive at unassailable conclusions.

Breast cancer is the most common cancer in the human female. The majority of cases occur in women over forty. A genetic factor is apparently involved, since the incidence is 10–15 percent greater in families who have had such cancer, and it also tends to develop several years earlier in daughters of mothers who have had it. The risk is somewhat increased in women who have never been pregnant, never nursed, or have had a late menopause.

Breast cancer is uncommon in young women (whose estrogen stores are high). The incidence increases with age, when estrogen levels are declining. Some researchers regard this as evidence that estrogen protects against breast cancer. But cancer can develop as long as twenty or thirty years after a stimulus. Does this mean that estrogen is responsible, but the cancer just develops years later? No such conclusion can be drawn. It may just be that the aging cell is more prone to cancer than the young cell. *As long as the basic cause (or causes) of cancer remain unknown, all such reasoning will lack the conclusiveness of unquestioned scientific fact.*

Perhaps the most comforting fact is that the incidence of breast cancer has not increased during the past quarter century, during which time estrogens have been in general use. But then neither has the incidence declined. It is a puzzling subject. An interesting line of research which may add pieces to the complex jigsaw puzzle involves a study of the relationship of specific estrogens such as estradiol and estriol to breast cancer.

Although there's no proof that estrogen has any role in *causing* breast cancer, there are nonmalignant conditions of the breast that can be *aggravated* by estrogen, such as cystic disease (lumpy breasts). Many breast specialists advise omitting estrogen therapy in women with known cystic disease, and possibly in women with a family history of breast cancer. They also warn that estrogen may stimulate a preexisting breast cancer, and so it is particularly important to be sure the breasts are free of palpable tumors before starting such hormonal therapy. Periodic self-examination is important. So are periodic checkups by the physician.

Interestingly, women with fibrocystic breast disease may show improvement when given progesterone compounds. This has led to the concept of "balanced" estrogen-progesterone therapy, rather than estrogen alone, particularly if there are any breast disorders which tend to be aggravated by estrogen alone.

To add to the confusion about the relationship of estrogen to breast cancer, it has been found that in some cases estrogen actually has a beneficial effect on breast can cer, specifically in women five years or more postmenopausal, producing temporary remission in about 25 percent of patients, especially in cases where the tumor has spread.

Finally, there is some evidence that hormones (cyclic estrogen and progesterone) may actually be a protection against breast cancer, though much more work and time are needed to properly evaluate this.

Of all female cancers, cancer of the cervix (neck of the womb) is the most readily diagnosed. The "Pap" smear and regular gynecological checkups should have made this a largely preventable disease by now. But for reasons difficult to explain, most women do not avail themselves of such preventive measures.

The cervix is the one area of the female genital tract which is "open for inspection". Hence smears taken from this area are quite reliable and can be quickly followed up. A high percentage of cure results from the treatment of *early* cervical cancer.

The cervix appears to be less sensitive to estrogen than the lining of the womb or breasts. As with the breasts and uterine lining, only long-term, carefully controlled, mass studies can give an accurate answer as to the relationship (beneficial or not) between cervical cancer and hormones such as estrogen and progesterone.

Cancer of the ovary has its highest incidence between the ages of 55 and 65. There are many different pathologic types, some more malignant than others. It is not yet possible to say what effect prolonged estrogen and/or progesterone therapy will have on the progress of this disease.

One of the most discouraging features of ovarian cancer is the inability to detect it at an early stage by some simple test. The best means of detection remains periodic pelvic examination, which is one reason why older women should have such examinations at least twice a year.

Hormones and Cancer

No discussion of hormones would be complete without including the birth control pills, which utilize both estrogen and a potent progestin. Said the government appointed medical advisory committee to the FDA recently: "The oral contraceptives present society with problems unique in the history of human therapeutics. Never will so many people have taken such potent drugs voluntarily over such a protracted period for an objective other than the control of disease."

Another unique feature is that, unlike hormones for menopausal or postmenopausal women, millions of *young* women are taking estrogen (and progestin). Various potential risks from "the pill" have been debated for years, with no definite proof on either side. So far there has been no hint of rise in cancer of the breast or genital organs. And some investigators suggest that these hormones may offer some protection against cancer.

Knowledge of the potential long-term effects of estrogen-progestin compounds requires much longer clinical experience under properly controlled conditions of observation and follow-up. Only such studies can conclusively answer the question as to whether the prolonged use of hormonal contraception will affect, either favorably or unfavorably, the incidence of breast and genital cancer.

※

6

Estrogen Replacement
Therapy

The beginning of health is to know the disease
CERVANTES

Ours is the most personal branch of medicine. The gyne-cologist-obstetrician, more than any other specialist, is truly a personal physician. In recent years patients have been turning to him with a request for pills—to keep them from aging or to make them young again.

Many women are now asking to have their "estrogen level" checked, as though it were oil for an engine. The implication is that a physician need only raise the level in order to erase complaints as well as wrinkles.

It isn't that simple.

I cannot subscribe to the idea that a woman's "femininity" should be rated according to the "percentage of superficial cells in the vaginal smear". I have found such smears quite limited in practical value. Nor can I agree with the concept that the doctor should treat "primarily and principally the vaginal smear, not the symptoms". There is already a tendency among women to confuse estrogen levels with sex appeal.

To understand hormone therapy, let's see how it began. It was in 1847 that cellular changes in human vaginal secretions were first described. Many years later, when Drs. Stockard and Papanicolaou discovered changes in the vaginal smear during menstrual cycles (with sub-

51

sequent development of the technique by Papanicolaou)
the way was paved for modern hormonal cytology. Dr.
Papanicolaou ultimately developed the famous "Pap" test
upon which our present studies of cell structure are based.

Although the Papanicolaou staining method remains
an excellent laboratory technique, which also permits diagnosis of cellular abnormalities by the experienced cytopathologist, much simpler staining methods are available
for those who are primarily interested in *hormonal* function. In fact, those doctors who routinely do "wet smears"
—that is, simply placing a drop of vaginal secretion under
the microscope—can get much the same information with
no staining at all. But if a preserved smear is wanted, there
are simple stains that serve admirably, and take less than a
minute to prepare.

What, then, are the problems in interpreting vaginal
smears in relation to "estrogen levels?"

What is actually seen in the smear is not just an estrogen effect, but the end result of an interplay between estrogen and other body hormones.

During pregnancy, for example, the body is suffused
with tremendous quantities of estrogen. Yet the "maturation index" of the vaginal smear will often show a "low
estrogen effect!" The reason is that the large amount of
progesterone, also produced, counteracts the estrogen effect,
yet bears no relation to the actual amount of circulating
estrogen the woman has. This is also why women taking
birth control pills (which contain estrogen and progestins)
often fail to show a "good" estrogen level. The same is true
of a woman who happens to be on hormonal therapy containing some androgenic (male) hormone. Her resultant
estrogen effect will be altered, not because she isn't getting
enough estrogen, but because this interplay of hormones in
the body does not reflect her true estrogen level. The adrenal
glands also put out substances that tend to counterbalance
estrogen effect.

In women who are still menstruating, smears for estrogen content vary from day to day. Such content is usually optimal between the eleventh and fourteenth days of a 28-day cycle. However, in the irregularly menstruating or non-ovulating woman (most middle-aged women are in this category), there simply is no "optimal" day to take a smear. Since the estrogen level does fluctuate, a single smear taken at random is really of very little value.

Smears are not a dependable measure of the absolute level of estrogen in the body, especially when a single test is made. In fact, as one cytologist put it, "for the diagnostic evaluation of the individual case on an individual specimen, the index is a loss of time for both the cytopathologist and the clinician." The index may confuse rather than elucidate, since a single specimen may lead the clinician to make a diagnosis merely on the basis of the index. Serial smears would be more significant.

Moreover, even *postmenopausal* smears show a fluctuant pattern for some time before settling down. And, if not fluctuation, a persistence of considerable estrogenic activity has been found in many studies of postmenopausal smears.

Many *external* factors can also affect the smear. These include the particular portion of the vagina from which the smear is taken, the presence of vaginal infection or bleeding, recent coitus or douching, recent vaginal medication (especially an estrogenic cream or suppository), presence of prolapse (bulging) of the vaginal tissues, the degree of postmenopausal response of aging tissues, and even the taking of certain drugs such as digitalis for heart conditions or preparations for diabetes.

Moreover, any smear sent to the laboratory may be differently interpreted by different observers who screen the slides.

One must also add that there is no agreement among cytologists, endocrinologists or gynecologists as to what constitutes a "normal" estrogen level at any given time, particularly at and after the menopause.

Suppose one finds a *high* percentage of "superficial" cells (fully matured by estrogen) in a woman well past menopause who is taking no hormones. Does this mean that all is well? No. In such a case, the physician is alerted to the *possibility* of an estrogen-producing tumor in the patient, or a uterine cancer. Some researchers have not noted such a correlation, while others have pointed out that a high estrogen index in older women is more often associated with ingestion of certain drugs (for heart conditions or diabetes) than with uterine cancer. I recently saw a 68-year-old patient who on initial examination had a high estrogen level. She had not been receiving estrogen therapy, nor was she being treated for any medical condition. She was found to have an estrogen-producing tumor of the ovary.

I have not found any real correlation between vaginal smears and the relief of specific symptoms of the menopause. Others have also pointed out that "the symptoms and not the laboratory data . . . serve as more accurate criteria in determining the efficacy of therapy."

The smear is often greatly "improved" by therapy that has no appreciable effect on the symptoms. Conversely, there may be considerable symptomatic improvement by therapy, with only a slight change in the smear.

Giving estrogen to a patient whose symptoms are unrelated to estrogen deficiency can be disappointing. I have in mind, for example, Mrs. G., a tall, thin woman, rather lined and angular, and looking all of her 55 years. Married and the mother of two, she had had a hysterectomy eight years previously for fibroid tumors. However, her ovaries had not been removed. Her list of complaints was varied. She was irritable and depressed. Her joints ached with bursitis. Her skin was dry and her hair was thinning.

She had a moderately poor estrogen effect on her

smear, and I gave her a "therapeutic test" with estrogen. Several weeks later she reported that there was no improvement in her condition. She was disappointed and wondered if perhaps she was not getting enough hormone. The dosage was increased. Still there was no appreciable effect. I explained that hormonal therapy helps only those complaints that are related directly or indirectly to actual hormonal deficiency, and there were no longer signs of such deficiency in her case. Although her estrogen smear was improved, *she* was not.

In another patient I found a "poor" estrogen smear but no symptoms. Mrs. S. was a small, plump woman who looked less than her 48 years. She was married and the mother of two children. She had gone through the menopause four years previously and she now came to the office for a checkup.

Her physical examination proved entirely negative. Her blood pressure was normal. The vaginal smear did show a low index of estrogen activity. However there was no appreciable thinning of the vaginal mucosa. She had no complaints, in fact felt quite well. I told her there was no specific need for any hormonal therapy at this time, and suggested that she check again in six months, or sooner if she had any discomforts.

The vaginal smear for estrogen activity has many limitations. It is seldom useful as an indication for therapy, except in cases of atrophic vaginal states. And it does not reflect "femininity."

Smears are more useful as a progression or regression *trend* (especially during prolonged therapy) than as indicators as to whether or not treatment is needed. In all instances, I have found that the patient's *symptoms* offer the most reliable guide both for the institution of therapy and regulation of dosage.

It would probably be more useful if laboratories reported "slight," "moderate" or "good" estrogen effect,

"compatible with the patient's age and time of cycle",
rather than attempting to give percentages, which can be so
misleading.

To advise specific therapy sight unseen, of course,
would be presumptuous. No one can direct what should be
done without proper examination.

Much depends on *what* is being treated. Only your
own doctor can decide whether hormonal replacement is
necessary, on what basis and for how long. This may even
include "preventive" considerations. There are many ways
to handle given symptoms, and your doctor has many drugs
at his disposal. The choice of drugs is particularly wide
when it comes to therapy for menopause. A long list of estrogenic and other hormones is available, not to mention
tranquilizers, sedatives, and a variety of other drugs. Most
hormones are so effective when taken by mouth that it is
rarely necessary to give injections.

Let us suppose you come to a gynecologist for a
checkup. It is your first visit and you are somewhat appre-
hensive. The first thing he will want to do is to take your
complete history. How old are you? Are you married? Do
you have children? How old are they? Have you had any serious illnesses? Any surgery? What about your periods? Are
they regular? If not, when was your last one?

Then he will ask about specific complaints. Does anything aggravate a particular symptom or relieve it? Do your
symptoms interfere with ordinary activity or with sleep?

He is likely to explore your family situation to see
what bearing it has on your symptoms. He will want to
know how well you get along with your husband, how you
deal with your children, whether you have any specific family or marital problems. He will inquire also into your oc-
cupation, your interests and finally your emotional problems.

You will then be prepared for a physical examination.

A specimen of your urine is examined. He will take your blood pressure. He will examine your breasts for lumps, palpate your abdomen and give you a pelvic examination and a "Pap" smear.

If you have no complaints and there are no objective findings of hormonal deficiency, no therapy is needed. However, if there are symptoms that suggest estrogen deficiency and there are no contraindications to hormonal therapy, I usually give a "therapeutic test" with estrogen. I tell my patient that *should* her symptoms be due to estrogen deficiency, she may expect relief. But if the symptoms are not due to such deficiency they cannot be expected to improve.

Here, for example, is a case showing what happens when some, but not all, of a woman's symptoms are estrogen-related. Mrs. B. is a woman of medium height with graying hair. She is 49, married with three children, and she enumerates a series of complaints that have plagued her since her menopause three years ago. She is tired and forgetful. Her heartbeat is fast. She can't sleep. She is troubled by hot flashes. Her breasts sag and she has lost all interest in sex.

After a few weeks of gradually increasing estrogen dosage, she reports that her flushes have completely disappeared, she is sleeping ever so much better, her palpitations have improved considerably, and her fatigue has lessened. However, her memory lapses remain unchanged, her breasts have remained flabby and she is still just as uninterested in sex.

Naturally she had hoped that *all* her complaints would be relieved. I explained that not all were necessarily due to one cause. Since she felt so much better, however, she was pleased.

Sometimes estrogen can relieve a nondeficiency symptom by a psychological effect. Mrs. C. was 48, married, childless. She complained of fatigue; she was depressed; her memory was weak. "I would like to be more youthful," she said, "with more zest and spirit."

Her physical examination was negative except for marked dryness and thinning of the vagina. When I found this condition, I asked whether she found intercourse painful. She replied that she rarely had intercourse because of marital problems with her husband.

I prescribed local estrogen to prevent the irritation that usually develops when vaginal tissues are so thinned. In addition I prescribed estrogen replacement therapy by mouth.

Three weeks later, she reported that she felt much stronger, more energetic and youthful. Her complaints were originally phrased in a way that made me feel that she was quoting some article she'd read on estrogen replacement therapy. She was evidently in a proper frame of mind to respond, judging by the speed with which she became "more youthful". Actually, her symptoms (except for the vaginal thinning) were not estrogen-related. They soon returned, in spite of continued estrogen with even higher doses.

Frequently when a placebo or mild sedative is prescribed instead of hormones, a woman's initial enthusiasm will result in great initial success. In this case, the pychological effect resulted from actual hormones.

Urinary symptoms can also be related to estrogen deficiency.

Mrs. H. came to the office with this complaint. A handsome, white-haired woman of 53, smartly dressed, she had become widowed after a long and happy marriage, and had recently remarried. Her menopause was five years in the past. Recently she was troubled by more frequent urination, including the necessity to get up at night to void, and she was aware of discomfort in the vaginal area during intercourse. The general examination proved negative but she did have a marked thinning of her vaginal tissues.

Now, the dividing line between the upper vaginal wall and the bladder is at best very thin. Therefore, when there is further thinning of vaginal tissues due to estrogen lack, it is not surprising that pressure upon the sensitive bladder area (as with intercourse) should cause discomfort. Moreover, the urethra and part of the bladder lining may become atrophic from estrogen deficiency, the same as the vaginal tissues. These urinary structures respond nicely to estrogen, and symptoms such as urinary frequency and painful urination are relieved *if* the sole cause of the symptoms is mucosal atrophy. However, urinary symptoms may also be due to other causes such as bacterial infection (cystitis) in which case the lack of response to estrogen requires further investigation. In this particular case, the local therapy alone relieved the patient's complaint.

In another case, the woman had both urinary and general complaints. I prescribed an oral estrogen and estrogen vaginal cream, the latter for immediate local effect on the tissues. The urinary symptoms gradually subsided, as did her other complaints.

Each doctor has his own way of handling his patients. No method is the only "correct" one. I prefer to give estrogen in cyclic fashion, at least at the start. I ask the patient to make a careful note of her symptoms and then to keep a record of the effect of estrogen therapy on those symptoms. If, within two weeks, there is no appreciable effect, I usually increase the dose enough to establish adequacy of the therapeutic test. I encourage my patient to call at intervals of three or four weeks, at which time I record on her chart her progress. Both benefits and any annoying side effects are recorded.

The dosage and choice of drugs is flexible and depends entirely on the woman's clinical response. I treat the symptoms, not the smear. I maintain a patient on the dosage that relieves her symptoms with minimal or no side effects. If none of her symptoms is relieved despite high dosage, I conclude that the complaints are not related to a lack of estrogen. In such event, the symptoms must be further investigated, for she naturally wants relief *no matter what the origin.*

Often the patient has many symptoms. A therapeutic test with estrogen may result in a complete elimination of perhaps three of the complaints, yet have no appreciable effect on the others. Thus there is a dramatic separation of estrogen-related and non-related symptoms. Insomnia, for instance, may be improved by the elimination of night sweats. Or the patient may continue to suffer restless nights because of financial worries or illness in her family. It is probable, too, that anxiety-like symptoms are often due more to fear of growing old than to hormonal factors. Then estrogens cannot be expected to alter or reverse such symptoms. It is difficult for a doctor to pigeonhole symptoms.

Take a woman who is depressed. Even if she is suffering from an estrogen deficiency, her depression may be unrelated to this lack of hormone. Depression is a symptom that can be present in women of all ages. Some causes are obvious. But I am convinced there is also a menopausal, estrogen-related depression, for it clears dramatically with estrogen replacement, is unaffected by a placebo, and returns if estrogen is discontinued. Such depressions are almost impossible to distinguish from the nonmenopausal depressions in middle-aged women. The elimination of other estrogen-related symptoms usually results in some improvement of the depression, but primarily because the woman feels generally better and is able to cope with some of her other problems. The depression remains, if to a lesser extent, and the roots may often be found in an exploration of her family life.

Many women are obviously in need of estrogen replacement but are so afraid of "hormones" that it requires a good deal of explanation to persuade them that estrogen does not cause cancer and may, on the contrary, make them feel much better. Others ask about therapy, yet are worried about side effects. Still others, who are given estrogen replacement for particular needs, clearly require a lot of "homework" in other areas pertaining to general health— for example, to lose weight, reduce smoking, or increase physical activity.

I give progesterone under specific circumstances. Normally, progesterone causes a shedding of the uterine lining, that is, menstruation. I find it useful for a patient who is not quite menopausal—that is, she is still having irregular periods. Such a woman is apt to be more in need of progesterone than estrogen, and I give both hormones, which serve to regulate her cycle.

However, if she has missed one or two periods and on examination is found to have abundant clear cervical mucus, it means she has *too much* estrogen and will probably have a whopping heavy period soon. Progesterone, given without delay, encourages a more normal, controlled menstrual flow.

Some physicians like to add testosterone (the male hormone) to estrogen therapy, supposedly to counteract some of the unpleasant effects of estrogen, and perhaps give a greater sense of well-being. However, I have found testosterone to be of rather limited value in middle-aged women, though of great value in younger women with premenstrual tension or painful periods.

Irregular, unexpected bleeding *as a result of therapy* can be a nuisance. Mrs. P. was 57, married, with no children. Her periods had stopped two years ago and she was suffering from flushes, headaches, depression and weight gain. I found nothing wrong with her physically except for a moderate estrogen deficiency. Estrogen therapy soon relieved her symptoms. But within a few weeks she was having irregular bleeding. I stopped the estrogen but the bleeding persisted. A curettage disclosed a tendency for the uterine lining to pile up. She was given a combination of estrogen and progesterone, and the uterine lining was "shed" every six to eight weeks. To date there has been no recurrence of irregular bleeding. For the past year, periods have been "scheduled" at six month intervals.

Bleeding or spotting as the result of estrogen therapy is not uncommon, but it usually shows up at an expected time—during the interval that estrogen is withdrawn for a week or so. If bleeding occurs at other times, such as while the patient is taking the pills, or if it persists for more than two weeks after therapy has been stopped, then it is necessary to look for organic causes. This usually means a curettage (scraping) of the uterine lining, often including a specimen from the cervix. A curettage is a minor hospital procedure.

The sensitivity of different women to estrogen varies. In general older women are more sensitive to any given drug than younger ones. An example is Mrs. E., a stocky, dark-haired woman of 54. She was widowed and childless, and her menopause was seven years ago. She was plagued by flushes and vaginal itching. I found a marked estrogen deficiency and gave her estrogen by mouth concomitantly with a local vaginal cream. Within two weeks her symptoms disappeared. However at that point she began to have light vaginal staining. This ceased when the medication was stopped. I then prescribed a lower estrogen dose, and the staining has not recurred. Regulating the dosage for each woman is necessary. It is important to find the optimal dose to bring relief of symptoms with fewest side effects.

Women who are past menopause are not usually pleased about the idea of menstruating regularly again. There is no need to insist on producing regular periods, unless some special reason (such as tendency to staining from medication) calls for it. Even then, it is usually possible to work out a schedule where the uterine lining is "shed" only once or twice a year. (Of course, women who have had a hysterectomy can have no vaginal bleeding problems.)

I also find progesterone useful for patients who need estrogen replacement but have a tendency toward lumpy breasts. Progesterone acts as an antagonist to unopposed estrogen. If this doesn't bring the desired results, I stop the estrogen altogether.

Such cystic disease of the breasts is normally uncommon after the menopause. An example is one of my patients, a fair-headed plump woman of 44. Married, with two active adolescent children, Mrs. D. had had no periods since her hysterectomy for fibroids two years previously. Her complaints included fatigue, an irritable disposition, restlessness, depression, and a tendency to perspire.

Since estrogen deficiency was suspected, this hormone was prescribed. Within the next few weeks her estrogen smear was distinctly improved. But she was not! All her symptoms were essentially unchanged, indicating that her complaints were unrelated to estrogen lack. Moreover, at her return visit I found several cystic areas in both breasts, which I had not felt previously. In fact, she herself had noticed them on self-examination. Aspiration of the fluid from the largest cyst revealed just clear fluid. She was advised to diminish her salt intake and to apply heat to the breasts when bathing. The cysts have gradually disappeared and, two months later, x-ray of the breasts revealed no unusual features.

Estrogen therapy definitely didn't help Mrs. D. But in other cases, where there *is* definite benefit from estrogen replacement, the effect upon sensitive breasts may be minimized by using smaller doses, as well as by the periodic use of progesterone to prevent unopposed estrogen stimulation of breast tissue.

Many women ask how long estrogen replacement

therapy may be kept up if there are beneficial effects and no annoyances.

Years ago, I used to discontinue such treatment after a few months. Often the patient continued to feel well. Sometimes she began to feel poorly again.

Today, I am in no rush to stop, particularly when a patient shows a tendency toward high blood pressure or signs of bone thinning. Since patients on estrogen replacement therapy are scheduled for checkups and "Pap" smears at regular intervals, it is a simple matter to reevaluate the needs each time.

7

The Estrogen Debate

A woman's always younger than a man of equal years
ELIZABETH BARRETT BROWNING

℘

A century ago medical science was ill-prepared to deal with menopause. For common menopausal problems, one physician in 1870 recommended, "Rest, reclining in the recumbent posture, with the feet higher than the pelvis, belladonna and opium suppositories . . . the ordinary tonics, and nervine tonics like arsenic and strychnia, change of habits and of scene."

Yet in the early 1930's, when endocrinology was still in its infancy, there were those who voiced strong objection to the way menopausal problems were being neglected, or, at best, treated as a stepchild.

Nobody can complain that the subject is neglected today. There is hardly a ladies' magazine that does not feature at least one article every few months on the subject. These often have been the source of confusion. But this is also true of *medical* articles.

At one extreme are the ultraconservatives who tell us: "Except in a minority of carefully selected cases, there is little more justification for giving drugs (including hormones) for the flushes and tantrums of the climacteric than there is for the blushes and waywardness of adolescence." Even though estrogen offers "immediate and dramatic benefit to the sufferer from climacteric symptoms, it should be adopted only as a last resort."

Regarding hormones, another writer states: "The object should be to reduce the symptoms to a point where they can be tolerated, rather than to remove them altogether."

One writer objects to the analogy of estrogen deficiency to thyroid deficiency or to eyesight problems, pointing out that "in all these deficiencies there are many lesser degrees which neither require nor receive treatment." He also asks why, if estrogen is so specific, do some report greater relief when estrogens are combined with other drugs such as tranquilizers, and points out that some emotional states may be worsened by estrogen therapy. His own study showed a significant percentage of improvement in menopausal symptoms by the use of a nonhormonal preparation.

The conservative *Medical Letter* which goes to doctors states that for obvious discomforts estrogens are "relatively harmless" if given "for a few months or a year or two at the most, and may be helpful for emotional distress."

Some feel that the *only* valid criteria for giving hormones at the menopause are flushes and sweats.

At the other extreme are those who advocate estrogens "from puberty to the grave" to maintain a certain numerical level on vaginal smear. There are a growing number of others, who are strong proponents of active intervention and long-term therapy. They term menopause a deficiency disease, and the woman a physiological castrate.

Finally, there are the vast majority—the moderates who are on the fence. They do not want to be coerced into a position which has yet to be proven. Many feel that hormones are being indiscriminately prescribed for many symptoms erroneously ascribed to change of life, that the pendulum has swung from undertreatment to overtreatment, and that the personal views of some authors are presented with such autocratic finality as to appear as unassailable fact.

The Estrogen Debate

Some doctors prescribe estrogen reluctantly. One reason, it seems to me, is that they believe many symptoms are unrelated to estrogen deficiency. In such cases, of course, treatment is discouraging and unrewarding.

Historically, and too often hysterically, estrogens have been endowed with malignant potentialities. Paradoxically, it has been pointed out that even conservative physicians may not hesitate to give sedatives or tranquilizers, yet they stop at the suggestion of estrogen replacement therapy. This is baffling to a good many doctors. Laments one endocrinologist, "Why it should be more natural physiologically to give a sedative than a natural hormone which the body produces is beyond me."

The attitude that "time will tide the patient over" seems to me regrettable, even if symptoms are not too severe. Sometimes moderate or even mild menopausal symptoms, superimposed on the other nonmenopausal symptoms, may create a heavier burden than a woman can comfortably bear. The point is that if during those few months her symptoms are disagreeable enough, both she and her family needlessly suffer.

Even though estrogens cannot cure emotional problems, a woman is better able to cope with these problems if her estrogen-related symptoms are relieved or eliminated.

An overworked doctor may not have time for a woman with menopausal problems. The treatment of menopause and postmenopause does take much time and much patience. As a result, some doctors may tell a patient, "Forget about it. Treatment merely postpones the inevitable."

This concept presupposes that no matter how long estrogen replacement therapy is given, the woman will get her "change of life" whenever therapy is stopped, just as though no treatment had been given. This is not necessarily true. Symptoms aren't apt to recur during long-term therapy or if treatment is tapered off gradually.

Some have said that the medical profession in the

United States, being male-dominated, is reluctant to treat the postmenopausal woman because of a subconscious anti-female feeling. This is nonsense. The entire training of a physician is geared toward the relief of suffering. It comes as no comfort to any doctor if he cannot help his patients. Besides, in countries such as Russia, where the majority of doctors are *women*, the treatment of the menopause is even more conservative than in our own. In my opinion, this has nothing to do with male-oriented or female-oriented medical professions.

Many doctors fear that a patient on hormonal medication will dose herself for long periods of time without supervision. They have seen ill effects from such self-treatment, and properly warn against it. Moreover, one has to be particularly careful in the case of elderly women whose memory span may be short. It helps in such cases to outline the instructions in writing or, in the case of the really aged, to inform a close relative of the instructions that go with the prescription. Patients should also call their doctor about any questions regarding symptoms, side effects or dosage. Self-medication can be minimized by the doctor who provides time limits on the renewal of prescriptions and insists on periodic checkups.

It is true that many women don't require any therapy and are not truly estrogen deficient. However this is of little comfort to those who *are* estrogen deficient and *would* benefit from therapy. It's like being reluctant to treat a patient with pneumonia because there are plenty of healthy people around. Yes, there are spry, 70-year-old women to be found in this generation. But there are also not so spry 50-year-old women who are in need of help.

Many patients themselves find the side effects of estrogen not worth the benefits. And some articles on estrogen replacement therapy describe benefits but fail to mention any of the possible drawbacks to such therapy.

Nausea is a common side effect. It is thought to be related to the nausea that occurs during pregnancy. Some estrogenic products have less of a tendency to cause this symptom than others. Nausea from estrogen generally diminishes the longer the drug is taken, and the tendency is minimized by taking the medication after meals.

Breast tenderness and swelling also are common, annoying side effects. Those women who suffered from cystic mastitis are particularly prone to develop this effect with continued therapy, and it can be most disconcerting. Others just have soreness of the breasts whenever they resume estrogen treatment, but no lumpiness. Decreasing the dose and the addition of progesterone minimizes the tendency to sore breasts.

Irregular, unexpected bleeding is a definite disadvantage of estrogen therapy, especially if its persistence necessitates a hospital curettage. Physicians have been so conditioned that any irregular bleeding, particularly in older women, is viewed with the greatest suspicion, and properly so. Is the bleeding due to estrogen? The only way to find out is to stop the medication. The bleeding will stop if due to the hormone. If bleeding does continue, a curettage is necessary. Since women differ greatly in their sensitivity to estrogens, it's often difficult to predict who will have this troublesome side effect. A few days' rest from therapy each month is designed to prevent build-up of the uterine lining and "breakthrough" bleeding.

One way to treat the problem of unexpected, irregular, hormonal bleeding is to cause the woman to menstruate according to a definite schedule by the use of progesterone. Many women would consider this a nuisance, but it may be the lesser of two inconveniences in those who have a persistent tendency to stain anyway. Besides, scheduled periods can often be planned for wide intervals, even several months apart.

Unfortunately, weight gain and swelling may occur from water retention due to estrogen administration. Salt restriction and diuretics may decrease this tendency. However, water retention is more hazardous in women with serious heart or kidney disease and for this reason estrogen is usually *not* given in such cases.

Estrogen promotes increased cervical secretion, occasionally to an annoying degree. While it may come as an unexpected change to the postmenopausal woman who has been used to the more abnormal state of "dryness", the vaginal secretion is actually more "normal" and is nonirritating. Furthermore, it may serve as a natural lubricant for sexual relations. In the rare case where it is persistently annoying, the secretions can be diminished by lowering the dosage or adding a progesterone product.

Estrogen therapy may cause darkening of the nipples and the area surrounding them, and discoloration around the face similar to the pigmentations of pregnancy. Sometimes a change in the brand of estrogen eliminates this tendency.

In general, the fear of growth of uterine fibroids in older women from the use of estrogens is exaggerated. Fibroids, benign fibro-muscular growths of the wall of the womb, tend to grow during reproductive life when estrogen output is greatest. They tend to "shrink" after menopause when estrogen levels are on the decline. It is not surprising, therefore, that some fibroids are stimulated to grow by the administration of estrogens. Much depends on the size of the fibroid tumors at the time estrogen therapy is contemplated. If they are already "borderline" in size, it would be preferable not to have any further enlargement. On the other hand, if the fibroids are relatively small, estrogen therapy may be given and the patient observed at more frequent intervals to make sure there is no rapid increase in size. Since fibroids may grow spontaneously, it is often difficult to assign a direct cause-and-effect relationship to hormonal therapy in the years before complete cessation of menses.

Finally, I should mention that the female sex hormones have important uses other than for the treatment of menopausal symptoms. Estrogen, for instance, has been used for painful menstrual periods; for irregular periods; for infertility cases to stimulate more favorable cervical secretions, to improve uterine growth and to stimulate the uterine lining; for stopping the too-rapid growth of young girls; for the treatment of acne; and even for the treatment of some cases of breast cancer. Estrogen has also been used as a possible preventive measure for osteoporosis and cardiac disorders. And, of course, birth control pills contain estrogen too.

Progesterone has been used in infertility cases whenever poor progesterone function is suspected. Sometimes it is used in cases of threatened, or repeated miscarriage, for irregular or heavy menstruation, to counteract an overproduction of estrogen, and for premenstrual tension.

Many young women taking birth control pills ask if such pills will prevent or postpone the menopause. The answer depends on how you define menopause. One who pioneered the development of the pill, Dr. John Rock, stated that although menopausal symptoms will often benefit from the pill, the pill can *not* postpone menopause "for menopause is the result of general aging, which is certainly not modified by the pill." The ovaries continue their aging process regardless of continued hormonal administration.

If, however, one defines menopause as the cessation of cyclic bleeding, then the contraceptive pill (or some other hormonal combination) *is* capable of continuing such artificial menstrual periods for an indefinite number of years, depending upon the product used and the dosage.

However, it seems to me that the important question is not whether the contraceptive pill *can* postpone menopause, but whether it *should* be used for this purpose. Contraceptive pills utilize not only estrogen but also a potent progestin (some products more than others). This accomplishes the primary purpose of the pill—effective contraception.

I prefer not to prescribe contraceptive pills into the middle and late forties. At *this age* irregular bleeding, which the pill may provoke, is looked upon with suspicion. When it occurs, the pills must be temporarily stopped and, of course, are then no protection against pregnancy. Besides, there is declining fertility at this age and it is not necessary to resort to the potent progestins contained in contraceptive pills. Some other means of contraception seems wiser. If a woman in her middle or late forties needs estrogen replacement, any one of a variety of estrogens will do. And if one wishes to induce artificial menstrual periods at intervals of one or more months, a natural progesterone is effective.

8

Beauty and Middle Age

Beauty is not caused, It is.
EMILY DICKINSON

❧

With middle age there often come certain changes in the appearance of a woman.

The hair, for instance, offers two main problems—too much in the wrong place, or too little in the right place. In the process of aging, many women are distressed to find some increase in hair, especially around the chin and upper lip. This tendency is influenced by familial factors and national origin. There is a greater tendency for such increased hair, even premenopausally, in women of Latin or Mediterranean background. In contrast, there is almost complete absence of such hair in oriental women of comparable age. In blonde Caucasians, extra hair is hardly visible.

Increased hair growth at the time of the menopause is considered physiological, similar to the hormonal shift at puberty and during pregnancy. Another cause of increased hair may be therapy with male hormones, which is why such hormones must be used cautiously, especially in women who already have a tendency to be hairy. Brunettes with oily skin are likely to be most sensitive. Fortunately, such effects of therapy can usually be reversed by stopping treatment.

Women often complain of hair thinning around the time of menopause. This is probably due to a relative increase in the amount of androgenic (male) hormone. The use of estrogens in the treatment of thinning, dull or drab hair in middle-aged women has been discussed from time to time. But there's no solid evidence indicating beneficial results. Clinically, some women report improvement in the appearance or texture of their hair when they're on estrogen replacement therapy. Just as many others report no change.

Of course, the most obvious hair change in the middle-aged woman is graying. Gray is not the presence of a new color, but rather the absence of pigment. Hair color is derived from pigment in the inner layer of the hair shaft. With gray or white hair, these cells contain only air. Why new hairs stop receiving this pigment is not known. (Incidentally, old hairs cannot suddenly "lose" their pigment, so hair does not "turn" gray.)

Estrogens or other hormones are of no value in stopping or reversing the graying process. In fact, one of the ads for estrogen replacement therapy frequently seen in medical journals shows a middle-aged woman with obviously gray hair.

A woman can either accept gray hair, hide it with a wig or color it.

She can do somewhat more about her skin.

Skin is a fascinating organ. It measures about 20 square feet, weighs about 7 pounds for women (10 for men), is self-repairing and, except in the case of children, self-cleaning. It protects the whole body against bacterial invasion and against loss of moisture. One square inch of skin contains about 15 feet of blood vessels which, by dilating and contracting, help regulate temperature. If a person is too warm, there are some 2 million sweat glands to help out, cooling by evaporation.

The skin has a rich network of nerves, but certain zones are "wired" for discomfort. For example, cold nerves are most numerous on the back, which is why dropping an ice cube there is not as humorous for the victim as for the onlooker. Heat nerves are most plentiful on the front of the body. "Touch" nerves are most numerous on the fingertips, which makes them especially sensitive. On the arm, the touch nerves are so sparse that if you touch yourself with two objects an inch apart, they will be perceived as one.

Our emotions show through the skin—pallor, blushing, sweating. And many sayings illustrate this relationship between skin and emotion—"I feel like jumping out of my skin," "He rubs me the wrong way," "He wants to save his own skin."

The face, particularly, mirrors emotion. Much of so-called premature wrinkling of the skin is probably due to repetitive facial expressions that have become habit. The woman who is constantly puzzled and worried is apt to have a furrowed brow simply because her facial expressions keep it that way. Similarly, wrinkling at the corners of the mouth are the trademark of the perpetually glum if the wrinkles slant downward, or of the perpetually smiling if they slant upward. There are other "happy wrinkles"—the little ones beside each eye, seen on those who are always smiling. The facial muscles under the skin, of course, are responsible for changes in expression, and the greater or lesser development of certain facial muscles will depend upon such repetitive expressions.

Voluntary changes of facial expression apparently do not leave creases as permanent as do repetitive, involuntary changes. If you stand before a mirror and register the facial emotions of astonishment, pain, delight or grief, they will not be as natural as those produced by spontaneous emotions. Anyone who has had to say "cheese" for a photograph knows this to be true.

Women often ask about "stretch marks" on the abdomen, especially after they become pregnant. Medically, these marks are known as "striae," or atrophic scarlike streaks. In French they are known as "whiplash marks."

Microscopically, they are truly "stretch marks" because there are less elastic fibers here. Many think that only pregnancy can produce such marks. This is not the only cause, nor do all pregnant women get them. They may also come from rapid weight gain, some debilitating diseases, and certain hormonal disorders involving the pituitary or adrenal glands. They have even been found in young male inductees, generally on the lower back, possibly due to a stressful situation causing excessive hormonal secretion in those who have a less resilient skin.

Not much can be done in the way of prevention or treatment of striae. There is more to say about tanning.

It is easy to understand the appeal of sunlight and tanning. Sunshine brings warmth, as well as the feeling of freedom that comes with shedding clothes. People equate a suntan with radiant health—"bronzed and fit". And in our society tanning has become a status symbol, a sign of wealth. Millions of men and women are willing to spend a good deal of money to lie for countless hours under the sun—a not-so-subtle form of masochism. First they lie on their backs till their eyes are dazzled. Then they turn over to study a rather uninteresting assortment of sand grains. The deeper the tan, the higher the status.

Unfortunately, such long and continued exposure actually ages the skin faster than anything else. Coarseness, drying, laxity and wrinkling are the main degenerative effects. Unexposed skin does not age nearly as rapidly as areas exposed to sun. The face and hands usually begin to show thinning and wrinkling long before the rest of the body.

All women long for a smooth, unblemished skin regardless of its color. It was probably always so. The ancient Greek Claudius Galen invented bleaches for freckles and the formula for cold cream still used today. Anti-wrinkle preparations over the centuries have been concocted from bread, incense, wax, turtle oils and what not.

76

It was only natural that our cosmetics industry expanded from merely covering up skin blemishes to fighting wrinkles. Various lotions and creams are peddled in an attempt to rejuvenate the skin. Russell Baker called this "the newest wrinkle in the youth game", or, "instant youth." One process for this involves proteins drawn from cow's blood to temporarily smooth and fill in furrows. The lotions are invisible because they react to light the same way human skin does. One application is said to cover up small wrinkles for about eight hours. The effect is always transient and, indeed, can vanish completely in a good rainstorm. And even the transient results are rather subjective. In one survey, about half the people asked guessed wrong about the side of her face on which a woman had put a wrinkle smoother. Nor does this product help neck wrinkles, which usually give away a woman's age. And, finally, some women feel a slight pulling sensation, a sort of tightness, from such products.

Various oily substances also have been applied to the face and body. These may be useful for lubrication, but will not prevent aging of the skin or wrinkles. Creams and lotions containing estrogenic hormone, too, have been marketed. The maximum amount of estrogen that the U.S. Food and Drug Administration permits in such products is 10,000 units per ounce. And this amount has no effect. Creams with a higher percentage of hormone, available on prescription, have given equivocal results. One observer claimed at least microscopic regenerative effect upon aging skin in five cases. (He also pointed out that a cream with a really high concentration of estrogen could cause atrophy of the skin).

Others have found the effect of ordinary hormonal creams to be both indefinite and inconsistent. The most that can be said is that there may be a little more hydration of the skin.

The same indefinite findings pertain to the effect on

the skin of estrogen taken by mouth or injection. Commenting on this subject, the *Medical Letter*, a report on therapeutics sent to physicians, says:

> Reports that estrogen administration restores or prolongs a youthful appearance or prevents or retards the effects of aging on the skin still await confirmation by controlled studies.

Many of the estrogens given in the form of birth control pills are combined with products having androgenic (male) properties. Some women taking these products complain that their skin is breaking out. Yet local or systemic estrogen is usually helpful for skin acne at any age.

Women are not put off easily. Perhaps it is true that in former days furrows and wrinkles were favored means of telling the future, something like palm reading. Today, they toll the future! So it is not surprising that plastic surgeons are concerned with the cure of wrinkles, the stigma of growing old.

One common procedure is the "face lift". An incision is made inside the hairline near the temple, and is continued down behind the ears to the nape of the neck. The sagging skin is then pulled to sufficient tautness to remove the wrinkles, yet retain facial mobility. The excess skin is cut, the incision stitched, and the face bandaged. The results may last for several years, or repeated lifts may be needed.

Another method is by dermabrasion—freezing of the skin and planing the surface with a rotary brush at speeds of 15,000 rpm. It has value, as well as limitations—all areas are not easily accessible.

Chemosurgery, chemical "face peeling" using a mixture of acid and phenol, has been used experimentally, primarily for supplementing the results of dermabrasion.

The process is painful. The skin becomes smooth and pink for six to twelve weeks, then gradually fades. The results are necessarily temporary, the changes of age recurring with time. Unfortunately, unscrupulous lay practitioners without proper training or experience have tried their hand at "quick chemical face lifts" and have scarred many women for life. To quote one medical article, "The setup is next to perfect for the unscrupulous person. He is dealing with a person who wants something desperately—youth . . . she is often willing to try even the most bizarre treatment . . . and if the result is not good, she is afraid to say anything because of the embarrassment of having friends know that she sought such treatments in the first place."

Another major problem confronting middle-aged women (and men, too, for that matter) is the tendency to gain weight, together with changes in the body shape, such as increased girth, and thicker arms and thighs.

No woman wants to bulge in the wrong places. Yet that's what begins to happen around the time of menopause. At first the fleshy changes are very subtle (Is she eating more?). Gradually, it becomes more and more difficult for her to hold the line and a feeling of resignation sets in. Reluctantly, she joins other middle-aged people with the same problem.

Why does this happen?

The stock accusation is: "You eat too much. Go on a diet."

The stock reply is: "I don't eat any more than I used to but I keep gaining."

Can it be that simple? Is it possible that millions of women all start eating too much at this time of life, and all develop the same type of figure problem? What an extraordinary coincidence!

And is it possible that all these women are inaccurate

in reporting their eating habits as being unchanged (even though their figures are changing)? Most curious. And their husbands seem to be involved in the same weight gain epidemic.

As it happens, recent evidence has shown that weight gain during middle age can occur on the same caloric intake that kept you trim in earlier years. In other words, what women report is true. It *does* take more effort to keep weight stationary at middle age. Just as it took more effort to hold the line during adolescence. Or during each pregnancy.

The truth of the matter is that there *is* a redistribution of fat during middle age. The problem is as vexing as it is mysterious. The average woman at this time of life begins to fill out in the waist, thighs, hips and upper arms. And scientists are not sure exactly why this happens. In fact, very little is known about the mechanism of fat distribution even in younger individuals. Take the pretty 18-year-old girl with a slim figure—except for "piano legs." Whatever the reason, it certainly isn't a calorie problem.

Is the "middle-age spread" due to menopause? To waning estrogen function? No, this weight redistribution is common in men, too, who apparently have no major hormonal shift at this age.

Giving estrogen replacement therapy has no slimming value whatever. On the contrary, it may lead to increased weight by causing fluid and salt retention. Many women taking birth control pills (which all contain estrogen) report difficulties maintaining their weight. Some of this is due to fluid retention, though other factors may play a role. For instance, when estrogen replacement therapy relieves menopausal symptoms, the feeling of well-being that results may be responsible for an increased appetite. Also pregnant women, who have a huge supply of estrogen, have a devil of a time controlling their weight.

So menopause *per se* is certainly not the cause of weight gain at this time of life.

Then is it something glandular? This is the cause that comes to mind whenever overweight is mentioned. Perhaps the first vision to enter the mind is an extreme, like the circus fat lady. There are, of course, glandular causes for obesity. But such cases are very much in the minority. Someone, in fact, commented that if any gland is involved it's the salivary one.

There's still a great deal to learn about the effect upon fatty tissue of such hormones as adrenaline, insulin and ACTH (adrenocorticotropic pituitary hormone). Even more fascinating are animal experiments showing that electrical stimulation of nerve centers on either side of the hypothalamus (the "center of emotions" at the base of the brain) can make an animal eat ravenously, whereas stimulation of other nuclei on the underside of the hypothalamus can make them lose their appetite. It's tempting to draw an analogy with compulsive eaters who say, with perhaps a great deal of truth, "It's my nerves."

The whole subject of fat conversion and storage is most interesting. We know, for example, that even in the absence of carbohydrate in the diet, as in an Eskimo diet, fat can be stored. So, there is no such thing as a "fattening" or a "non-fattening" food. Or a "reducing" food.

Nevertheless, calories do count. "Calorie" is a French word, derived from the Latin "calor" which means heat. A small calorie is the amount of energy needed to raise the temperature of one gram of water one degree centigrade. A large calorie will raise one thousand grams of water one degree. When food calories are mentioned, it is the large calories that are meant. Thus, one gram of carbohydrate or protein supplies four calories; one gram of fat furnishes nine calories.

In the process of aging, the need for calories decreases.

The same diet will result in weight gain at fifty that did not at thirty. Not because of age alone, of course. But this *is* one more variable influencing body requirement. Thus diet adjustment is desirable at this age.

Unfortunately, the average person is often taken in by "guaranteed to lose weight fast" schemes that do no credit to those who administer the services, as well as a lot of over-the-counter nonsense. To quote the director of the Department of Foods and Nutrition of the A.M.A., "The obese individual will learn that clinics promising 'get slim quick' are usually more interested in 'get rich quick' than they are in the welfare of the patient."

But every age has had its colorful and vociferous food faddists. One extremist in the vegetarian movement was Sylvester Graham (of cracker fame). He proclaimed that meat incited sex desires.

Probably the most remarkable faddist was "Professor" Arnold Ehret. In his book, *The Mucusless Diet Healing System,* he taught that:

> *Every disease,* no matter by what name it is known to Medical Science, is CONSTIPATION, a clogging up of the entire pipe system of the human body . . . The average person has as much as ten pounds of uneliminated feces in the bowels continually, poisoning the blood stream and the entire system. Think of it!

His cure? A fruit and nut diet. Aside from curing this universal ailment, his special diet was also supposed to help sterility and impotence.

What about exercise? Isn't lack of exercise—the sedentary life of the older individual—the basic cause of middle-age spread? While it's not really the cause, it is a small contributor. It's true that older people are generally less active. Some hardly do anything more strenuous than turn a television dial. And exercise unquestionably has many other benefits. However, let's not overestimate its role in weight reduction.

To work off a single milkshake, you'd have to walk for over an hour or swim for over a half hour. A hamburger takes an hour of walking or 45 minutes of bicycling to work off. With an hour of *hard* exercise daily you might lose about a pound of fat every ten days. So weight loss through exercise, without proper diet, is most difficult, especially if the activity increases your appetite. In addition, middle-aged people who lead sedentary lives should get their exercise gradually, rather than in spasmodic bouts of strenuous activity.

How to lose weight without really trying? You can't. But there are certain helpful suggestions. You should have a medical examination to determine what may be contributing to obesity and whether there is anything physically wrong that may interfere with a dietary regimen. Forget about prescribing your own diet for weight control. A short-term diet will *not* solve your problem. A complete change of eating habits is required. In most cases, if you lose a pound a week, the diet isn't too strenuous, since it requires a daily food intake only five hundred calories below what you need to live and work.

In any event, if you should have a tendency to be overweight, at least you are probably blessed with a full bosom.

Throughout history, women have been most concerned with the appearance and care of their breasts.

There was a time when youthful contours were good enough. But today, in popular circles, sheer size seems to be the goal. Venus de Milo had a 37-inch bust, but the present cult of the bosom strives toward ever higher peaks. Standards are now being set by the well-endowed Hollywood stars. As if to out-distance all competition, one California cabaret performer achieved a 44-inch bosom by the surgical insertion of plastic material. Will someone try for 46 inches next year?

Actually, our preoccupation with bustlines is not new. Ancient folklore even endows the breast with hidden powers. According to Roman legend, our giant galaxy, the Milky Way, was formed by Hercules suckling at Juno's breast with such force that the milk spilled into the heavens. And many Roman wine cups were shaped to the dimensions of a particular mistress or famous personage such as Cleopatra or Helen of Troy. Since those days, artists and sculptors have depicted the breast in every possible shape and form.

The breasts also figured in cultural superstitions. The Chukchi of Siberia tabooed certain foods (like quail) to young women in the belief that the breasts would fail to develop. But most cultural and anthropological differences in the breasts were purposely created in accordance with what was considered beautiful. Among the Uganda of South Africa, for example, long, pendulous breasts were the ideal. From a very early age, nipples were greased and pulled and the breasts actually tied down. "The result was that they were soon able to fling the breast over their shoulder to feed the child carried on their backs." The Payagua "tie leather belts across the breasts of the young girls as soon as they have reached full natural development . . . thus, before the girls reach the age of 24, their breasts sag to their waists."

Don't laugh. Our own vogue of flattening the bosom in the flapper era gave rise to the Boyish Form Brassiere Company. They advertised a breast-constricting device to "give you that boy-like flat appearance".

In some cultures the breasts are exposed. This was true of the women of ancient Crete, as well as the women of many African tribes today.

Climate and national origin also seem to influence the

shape of the breasts. Women living in very cold climates supposedly retain their youthful appearance longer than those in hot climates.

And probably it's always been true that few women think their breasts are just right. Or, if they are right one year, next year's fashion cycle may change matters.

Most complaints about breast changes come from women themselves, not from their husbands. Psychiatrists tell us that men like breasts, perhaps because their earliest memories of warmth, comfort and sympathy came from the maternal bosom.

In middle age, a woman may find that there is an increase in fat that makes her breasts fuller. But, as she grows older, breast and fat tissue decrease and flabbiness is often the result. To develop breasts, women resort to an endless variety of remedies—cream, lotion, massage, exercise, vibrating machines and vitamins. None has any effect on the size and shape of the bosom.

The fact is that the breast is composed of milk-producing tissue, supporting fibrous tissue, and fat; there are no muscular elements at all. Therefore no muscular exercise can develop the bust, except to increase the girth of the whole chest. Neither will massage or vibrating machines cause any change in size.

The advent of birth control pills, with their estrogens and progestins, probably did more for the female breasts than all the other methods combined. Although one pill manufacturer is supposed to have quipped that there is no link between birth control pills and bust inflation, the national average bra size reportedly has changed from 34B to 36B. Actually, though, the pills produce only a transient increase in breast size by promoting fluid retention everywhere, including the bust. This is a desirable "side effect" for small-breasted women, but the effect is gone once the pills are stopped. And at no time is there any real increase in the amount of breast tissue itself. Most women with normal menstrual cycles experience this transient, some-times painful enlargement of the breasts premenstrually each month.

The postmenopausal woman whose breasts have be-come somewhat flabby and smaller will often ask whether estrogen replacement therapy will improve her figure. The answer is that estrogen (with or without progesterone) will temporarily increase fluid retention and make the breasts feel and look a little fuller while on therapy. The effect, however, is not as marked as in younger women, since the postmenopausal breast is generally less sensitive to estro-gen.

The only permanent way to increase or decrease the size of the breasts is by plastic surgery. Surgical attempts at breast enlargement go back forty years or more, when surgeons tried grafting fat from the buttocks and inserting this fat between the breasts and the chest wall. The results were almost uniformly poor. In the first place, most flat-chested women don't have much to spare from their but-tocks. Furthermore, the buttock incision, besides leaving a scar, left a depressed area—a rather large dimple where it wasn't wanted. Also, transplanted fat becomes absorbed to an extent that, in time, almost nullifies the original intent.

About fifteen years ago, surgeons tried inserting a plastic sponge but this shrank in time, became hard and often painful because of infiltration of scar tissue, and often had to be removed.

Then came silicones. These are man-made substances derived from quartz (silica), synthesized into all sorts of rubbery and liquid forms. Some silicones are even con-tained in such items as automobile polish, hair sprays and shaving creams. It seemed only natural to explore the potential of these substances by injecting liquid silicones to augment body tissue. However, the initial enthusiasm for these injected materials began to subside following reports of undesirable reactions such as foreign-body granular lumps, which could not be distinguished from lumpiness that might be caused by a tumor. Furthermore, the material had a tendency to drift. The Food and Drug Administration, therefore, classified silicones for injection as "new drugs". Injection into the breasts, at least, is now illegal. Under FDA protocol, some investigators are testing the material in other body areas. Nevertheless, a black market of silicone injections is said to be flourishing, spurred by women demanding to be made ever larger by the "wonder filler".

More recently, a special silicone rubber implant has been developed which can be inserted *between* the chest wall and breast. The outer mold of silicone rubber cannot be invaded by scar tissue, and the inside is a soft gel that gives the breast a more normal consistency. Usually, though, it's firmer than natural breast tissue. In contrast to silicone injections, this type of implant does not go into the breast itself, but is placed under the breast by means of an incision at the base. Cosmetic results are generally good. Even so, many surgeons inform their patients that future discoveries may lead to the advisability of removing the implants, and require that their patients accept this possibility before undertaking the operation.

Every physician has had patients who complain about small breasts. Mrs. L. was 43, happily married and the mother of an adolescent girl. Menopause in her case had taken place six years ago from surgical removal of the uterus and ovaries for fibroids and cysts. Except for moderately atrophic vaginal tissues, her physical examination was negative. I explained to her that, although hormonal therapy could help her vaginal condition, no permanent changes in the size of her breasts could be expected. This is exactly what took place. Several weeks later, she reported improvement in her vaginal secretions but her bosom remained as it had been.

Another woman, before cosmetic surgery, had excessively large, pendulous breasts. She was married and, at 45, childless. Her periods were regular. Her chief complaint was weight gain. In her twenties, she had weighed about 135 pounds. For cosmetic reasons she had had plastic surgery to make her breasts smaller, and the result satisfied her. But, since then, she had gained about fifty pounds. Her breasts hadn't increased in proportion, and the imbalance between the size of her body and her bosom upset her. A physical examination showed there was nothing wrong with her except general obesity. She was put on a diet, but she didn't stick to it.

Excessively large, pendulous breasts do create problems. Plastic surgery is functional, as well as cosmetic, since huge breasts can cause posture problems, backaches and perspiration rashes. In fact, physiological studies have shown that very large breasts can even hinder breathing. The weight of a large breast is considerable, if all the blood and fluid it contains is taken into account.

In such cases, excess tissue is removed from each breast and the nipple is repositioned. As a medical student, I recall watching such an operation from the operating room balcony. The surgeon had removed the nipples, which had been carefully laid aside. He had also removed the excess breast tissue. Then, he turned to the nurse who was assisting him and said, "Left nipple, please." She froze. I could see her eyes widen in disbelief, as she realized that she had not kept track of which nipple came from which side. Then, as the surgeon's eyes began to twinkle, she gave a long sigh of relief as she realized that it really made no difference.

9

Sick at Heart

Hope is itself a species of happiness. . . .
SAMUEL JOHNSON

☙

Depression. The word itself has a melancholy sound. It is a down-in-the-dumps word without a single redeeming feature.

Being depressed is like thinking in a minor key. Why a minor key should be associated with sadness and a major key with brightness are musical mysteries yet to be solved. Sometimes both are found in the same piece. Bach liked to end a composition in a major key no matter what the previous mood. And Mozart was a master at skilful weaving between major and minor even within the same measure. Actually, there really is an association between music and medicine that dates back to Greek mythology. Apollo was the god of both music and health, and the Bible describes how King Saul's depression was helped by "little David" playing on his harp. In the seventeenth century, *The Anatomy of Melancholy* described music as an excellent remedy against despair that could "expel grief with mirth". About a century later, an English physician wrote that "music . . . allays the inordinate passion of grief and sorrow."

This "inordinate passion", it seems, becomes more common as one gets older. Nor is it surprising that depresion is a frequent complaint among women who have reached menopause and middle age.

Of course, sadness over such things as illness, loss of a job, or death of someone close is appropriate. Neurotic depression, on the other hand, is the kind that is inappropriate to one's surroundings—the birds are singing, yet you feel depressed; everyone in the family is in good health, but you're sad. As one patient said to me: "The way I used to feel premenstrually, that's how I feel all the time now."

Is depression caused by the hormonal changes of the menopause? The answer is yes and no. The fact is that *both* psychic and somatic influences may play a role, and one may even mimic the other. Some women with depression and estrogen deficiency report that a "cloud has lifted" upon correction of the deficiency. The relief is really quite dramatic. But other women with apparently similar complaints and findings report no effect, despite correction of the estrogen deficiency. Why?

Because depression, being only a symptom, has various causes. When unrelated to an existing estrogen deficiency, it is not surprising that replacement therapy fails to alleviate this symptom.

By way of analogy, let's consider another symptom—headache, and assume that in a particular woman the headache is caused by eye strain. Correction of the ocular problem will relieve the headache. But another woman, with headache *unrelated* to eye strain, will not be relieved of her headache by the prescription of new glasses, even though she may need the glasses to improve her vision.

Let's consider the relationship of depression to a lack of estrogens. There was Mrs. R, an attractive woman, but quiet and withdrawn. She was married and the mother of three children. Her last period had been five years before, when she was fifty. She suffered flushes and perspired a good deal; her hair was thinning, her skin dry, her breasts flabby. But what bothered her most was a sense of depression every morning.

"After a sleepless night, it all looks so hopeless," she said, sighing.

Since there was evidence of marked estrogen deficiency, estrogen therapy was begun. In the first two weeks there was only a slight improvement in the depression. The dose was increased and then she showed a marked improvement.

"The depression is gone," she reported. Two months later the news was even better. "I haven't felt so good in ages. No depression. For the first time in years, I sleep well."

In her case, she reported happily that estrogen therapy was "the greatest tranquilizer in the world."

Another patient, who was forty, married for the second time and one year past her menopause, was started on estrogen and progesterone therapy for depression. She also complained of sagging breasts and dull hair. After two weeks, she reported that as far as her depression was concerned, it was "as though a cloud had lifted". But then she reported that the depression had returned when she took progesterone, which was then stopped. Although there was no appreciable improvement in the condition of her hair and breasts, there was no recurrence of the depression. And she has been able to cope with her family problems much better.

When Miss C. came for her first visit, she complained of a tendency to burst into tears. After her physical examination, she was started on estrogen as a "therapeutic test" and within a few weeks the tendency to weep disappeared.

The type of crying spell associated with hormonal imbalance is usually described as "I cry for no reason". Because of this hormonal relationship, it is easier to treat, and improvement is often quite dramatic. But results are poor in depressions which are hormonally unrelated, as in the following case.

Mrs. T., a tall, attractive woman of 46, had her menopause two years before coming. She complained of flushes, insomnia, and depression for the past year. She showed a moderate estrogen deficiency. Estrogen therapy was given, with prompt relief of the flushes. The insomnia was also helped somewhat, since she was no longer awakened by the flushes. However, there was no effect at all upon her depression, despite considerably increased dosage. The depression evidently was unrelated to estrogen deficiency.

A woman who has reached menopause may have many other reasons to feel depressed *aside from hormonal deficiency.*

If she has been unable to have children, or has had fewer than she wanted, the menopause represents a vanishing hope, a closing of the door on what she may consider verification of her personal worth. In those cultures in which childbearing is crucial to a woman's self-concept, to remain childless often leads to despair unless other sources of creativity and self-esteem exist. In such women, the menopause is a stark reminder that the years are creeping up. In fact, *any* reminder that a woman is getting older is unpleasant.

A woman doesn't become someone else at the menopause. She is the same person as before. Moreover, her reactions to the physiological change will be determined largely by the type of person she always was; just as her entry into adulthood is influenced by her adolescent experiences and those, in turn, are influenced by her childhood ones. At each step, a woman meets life in terms of her own self-evaluation as a female. It is hardly surprising that those women who derive continued satisfaction and pleasure from their marriage, children and work feel much less threatened by "the changes" than those who don't.

Depression often is caused by an inability to cope with anger and aggression. Expression of aggression is usually discouraged in little girls ("it's not ladylike" or "don't be a 'tomboy'"). The repressed anger may be turned toward the self. The result is depression.

Sick at Heart

Some women become depressed at the menopause because they equate the loss of menstruation with loss of "femininity". Since the emotions are not unrelated to glandular function, one can speculate almost philosophically whether such feelings contribute to differences in the way women cease to menstruate—some abruptly, others falteringly as though to "hold on" as long as possible. But it is not that clear-cut. (In this connection, it has been suggested that unresolved conflicts may develop into a host of functional pelvic disorders in order to gain attention and sympathy from family and physician.)

Loss of physical attractiveness, however gradual, is tremendously depressing to many women, especially those who have always considered their looks their main asset. Nor do they derive any comfort from thumbing through those women's magazines which emphasize youth and glamor.

Depressing marital problems also frequently arise at this time of life. A husband may be busier than ever, perhaps more demanding, less understanding. And this may be coupled with a woman's anxiety about losing her husband's affection because she considers herself less attractive. This is even more depressing if a woman interprets her husband's gradually diminishing sexual interest as an indication that she means less to him. In addition, many women erroneously believe that menopause means loss of their own capacity to enjoy sex.

Financial problems often plague a family at this time of life too, especially if several children reach college age simultaneously. Caught in a financial "middle age squeeze", many people in their forties and fifties find it increasingly difficult to make ends meet.

Anxiety about job security for the middle-aged working mother is another cause of unhappiness. If she is seeking outside employment to supplement the family income, she may meet with a good deal of bias. If she already has a job, she may fear replacement by someone younger. Or, if she becomes successfully immersed in full-time work outside the home, she may experience pangs of guilt about her primary responsibility—her family.

Yet women who have always been homemakers, who have remained in the kitchen, often experience a let-down when their children have grown. To such a woman, taking care of a household and children is on a level with a man's job; when it is taken away it seems to spell forced retirement. And for women with few outside interests, idleness and boredom are the depressing results.

If the children are still living at home, they are likely to be at an age when they themselves can be very trying: "Children are now tyrants, not the servants of their households. They contradict their parents, chatter before company, gobble up dainties at the table, cross their legs, and tyrannize over their teachers."

The quotation is not from a local newspaper, but from Socrates about 2,300 years ago. Times haven't changed much.

Shakespeare said, "I would there were no age between ten and three-and-twenty, or that youth would sleep out the rest; for there is nothing in the between but getting wenches with child, wronging the ancientry, stealing, fighting."

The sexual revolution of our era has made parents of adolescents particularly worried about sexual promiscuity, which has been called the "copulation explosion". This is the time when mothers, especially, tend to breast-beat and cry, "Where have I failed?" It is also a time when mothers themselves feel that they are going through the most difficult stage of their lives. At the time of the menopause the mother is often less able to cope with even routine family problems because her own emotional reserves are so low.

Yes, menopause comes at a bad time. In addition to

the discomforts of hormonal imbalance, a woman has reached a stage in life where she equates loss of menstruation with loss of attractiveness, health and self-esteem as a woman, and at the same time tends to magnify marital, financial and familial problems.

It is small wonder that depression is one of the most common complaints of middle-aged women.

One of the most common complaints I hear from my patients is their inability to sleep. It is estimated that perhaps one-third of the population suffers some degree of insomnia. The causes are almost without limit. Commonly cited are overstimulation, understimulation, overexertion, underexertion, high blood pressure, low blood pressure, a full stomach, an empty stomach, noise, heavy bedclothes, fears, anger, frustration, worries, anxieties and many others.

It's hard to believe that in this day and age the basic mechanism and purpose of sleep remain a mystery. All we can say for sure is that every living thing appears to require sleep—with possible rare exceptions. It is said that the nurse shark can swim for years without sleep, at least when observed in an aquarium. It may be, of course, that the shark sleeps while swimming, but it's a bit hazardous to observe the sleeping pattern at close hand.

Out of 24 hours, a human infant will sleep for 21; at 6 months he will sleep for 18, and at one year of age for 15 hours. The requirements graduallly decrease until adolescence, at which time 6 to 8 hours are required. This figure is maintained more or less throughout life, so that by age 65 a person has slept away some 20 years.

Insomnia is especially common in the middle-aged woman. Menopausal women are apt to be awakened periodically with flushes and sweats. Or they toss and turn most of the night, fall asleep towards dawn and are exhausted the rest of the day. The early morning riser may have a depressive illness; the fitful sleeper may suffer anxiety; and those who have trouble falling asleep are often plagued by tension, resentment and frustrations.

Nothing gives me greater satisfaction than to help a patient overcome her sleeplessness. Often estrogen therapy helps dramatically, and a woman reports happily that she is "sleeping like a baby". But this is not to say that estrogen always helps insomnia. When sleeplessness is completely unrelated to hormonal deficiency, no benefit may be expected from such therapy.

Like insomnia, fatigue is often characteristic of both middle age and the menopause. Some women report greater vigor with estrogen therapy. Yet there are many instances where fatigue is completely unrelated to hormonal deficiency. When Mrs. S. came to me, she told me that her chief problem was fatigue. She was 59 and had had her last period 7 years previously. Divorced for 18 years, she had one grown son. Her job, in a dress shop, was frustrating. She worked long hours. She smoked two packs of cigarettes a day. She hadn't had a vacation in years.

She had been taking an adequate amount of estrogen for the past 6 years. It seemed to me that the target of her dissatisfaction was her work rather than her body.

There was no sign of estrogen deficiency. I suggested that she take a vacation; she was to continue her estrogen dosage as before. She said anxiously that it would be impossible for her to get time off. But I persuaded her to go, and a month later she called to say her fatigue had disappeared.

Often the opposite is true—the less you do the more tired you are. Since mature women often have too much leisure and are bored, they complain of exactly the same "exhaustion" as the overworked mother.

In that case I usually ask, "What are you tired of? Exactly what would you do if you weren't so tired?" The answer to such questions sheds light on the woman's home situation, her personal interests and her emotional state.

The children of middle-aged women are relatively independent. They may have left for college. They may be married. The woman feels less needed, literally let down. She has too much leisure and doesn't know how to fill the void. Sometimes the complaint, "I'm tired," really means "I'm tired of what I am doing." Or, more correctly, "I'm tired of what I am *not* doing . . . I'm tired of my way of life."

So a common cause of chronic fatigue is plain boredom. A woman suffering from boredom is just as weary as the overworked woman. But the cause is emotional and the symptom is produced by her being in a continuous state of tension. To tell a bored woman to get more rest makes no sense.

Once I was taken aback by the initial request of a new patient. "I want a 'Pep' smear," the woman said as I was taking her history. I hesitated a moment, since the dialect didn't seem to fit her.

"You mean 'Pap' smear," I said, referring to the familiar vaginal smear named after its originator, Dr. Papanicolaou.

"No, a 'Pep' smear," she repeated, "to see if I need hormones to pep me up." The woman was going through "the changes", and fatigue was one of her chief complaints. She was also having moderate flushes and slept poorly.

Is there a relationship between menopause and fatigue? There is, but an indirect one. When estrogen is given to women who have signs and symptoms of a definite estrogen deficiency, they feel better. If flushes or night sweats are eliminated and sleep becomes undisturbed, naturally there will be less fatigue. And while hormones cannot solve such problems as boredom or emotional conflicts, the treated woman is better able to face those prob-

97

lems. On the other hand, if there is no deficiency of estrogen manifested by symptoms or signs, or even by "Pep" smears, hormones cannot be expected to benefit fatigue.

One of the most frequent questions a fatigue sufferer asks is whether vitamins are needed. Very seldom. The same is true of thyroid medication, which should be based on actual need, as determined by tests, rather than on the vague complaint of fatigue. And that goes for iron too, though anemia should always be checked for when fatigue is a chronic complaint.

As for "mood lifters" such as amphetamines, they may bring about a temporary artificial lift but there are many undesirable side effects, and the roots of the problem still remain.

If a complete physical examination is negative, and if there is no iron, thyroid or hormonal deficiency, or if such deficiency has been found but corrected while the complaint of fatigue persists, psychological help is probably necessary.

Another troublesome problem at this time of life is headache. You can consult a doctor in each of a half dozen different specialties for your headache, and each one would consider it quite possible that the cause lies within his own field. The eye man will look for refractive errors, the ear-nose-and-throat specialist will check the sinuses, the allergist will start investigating sensitivities to dust or pollen, the psychiatrist will consider hidden emotional conflicts, the gastroenterologist will ask about your diet, the proctologist will wonder why you came, and the gynecologist or endocrinologist will consider hormonal deficiency.

That is to say headache, the most common of all physical discomforts, has many possible origins.

It is believed that by far the commonest type, constituting perhaps 90 percent, is the so-called vascular headache—dilatation of the cranial arteries, mainly branches of the large neck arteries. Everyday stresses seem to contribute significantly. In women, resentments, dissatisfaction, domestic and social difficulties and fear of illness are common precipitating causes. Migraine headaches tend to be intermittent, with intensification during a menstrual period.

Very anxious people often seem to think of brain tumor first when they get severe headaches. Fortunately, this is a rare cause. Other, more common organic causes include ocular and sinus disorders. The mere quality or location of the pain should not be used to conclude that a headache is of emotional origin, or else organic causes may be overlooked. Also not to be overlooked is the fact that headache can be caused by drugs—any drug.

Headache was probably common back in ancient times. Apparently primitives used sharpened stones to drill holes in the skull to let out evil spirits. The ancient Greeks used the bark of a willow tree as a favorite headache remedy. Various African tribes used roots, spells and incantations. In the Middle Ages, bleeding patients with leeches was a standard treatment for headache, as well as for every other common ailment. And liquor, of course, has always been used as a pain killer.

Aspirin, discovered in 1899, remains the most popular analgesic in every part of the world. Americans alone consume about forty tons of aspirin a day. Two aspirins give an optimal effect—that is, taking more than two at a time has no advantage. Giving a combination of several pain-killing drugs does not have an additive effect, contrary to popular belief. What you get is the effect of the strongest ingredient. Caffeine is sometimes added, and may be of value in constricting the cerebral blood vessels, especially in tension headache. Ergotamine tartrate is useful in migraine.

Inevitably, middle-aged women near or after menopause wonder whether headache is one of the symptoms of hormonal deficiency. It is certainly a common symptom of women at this time of life, and it is not difficult to see how the alleviation of some of the other complaints related to hormonal deficiency can also have a beneficial effect upon headache. For example, a woman whose flushes and night sweats are relieved, who consequently sleeps better and feels better, will probably experience headaches less often. There are many factors involved, and it is entirely possible that headache, like fatigue, will be indirectly helped by estrogen replacement. But not necessarily more than by an analgesic. Or a placebo.

Obviously, if headache in a middle-aged woman is caused by such factors as stress, boredom, too much responsibility, too little responsibility, fears, anger or a multiplicity of other factors, the administration of estrogen can at best be of only indirect benefit.

There are some cases in clinical practice where headache is dramatically relieved specifically by estrogen replacement. And if the woman responds that way to estrogen alone, I believe the hormonal medication should be continued. But attributing a cause-and-effect relationship must await large-scale, controlled studies.

10

To Be a Woman

The modern woman has generally regarded menstruation as a necessary nuisance. It is called by various names, depending on one's attitude. If it happens to be painful, it is likely to be called "the curse"—a term not unlike the primitive "possessed by demons". A somewhat kinder referral is "being unwell," which implies an element of illness. What is often meant by "unwell" is that the few days prior to each menstrual period may be accompanied by a miserable set of symptoms known as the premenstrual tension syndrome.

In fact, menstruation for some women means going through the "changes" every month.

Premenstrual tension is very common. Seventy percent of all women experience it, though many do not recognize it as such. Premenstrual tension has no respect for age until a woman finally stops ovulating and menstruating. One of the blessings of the menopause is the relief from this monthly emotional change that plagues so many for anywhere from two days to two weeks before each period.

In some European countries such as France and England, the pattern is even legally recognized by placing premenstrual tension in the same category as "temporary insanity". This means that women are considered less responsible for bizarre actions at this time of the monthly cycle.

The symptoms of premenstrual tension are bloating, headache, breast fullness and tenderness, swelling of the feet, weight gain, backache, abdominal discomfort, worsening of skin disorders, migraine, nervousness, change in libido, insomnia, irritability, poor concentration and general irascibility. The woman will often admit, "I'm not fit to live with." Any combination of these symptoms may be present. They are temporary and disappear with the onset of the menstrual period. I know of professional singers who avoid public appearances at this time of the cycle because impairment of voice from laryngeal congestion may also occur. In its most severe forms, premenstrual tension may lead to states of complete panic, or be a factor in crimes of passion or violence.

There are many theories as to the cause of premenstrual tension. One of the most plausible is that the symptoms are due to edema, which is water and salt retention. The emotional symptoms probably result from edema of the brain. There is some evidence that the severity of symptoms is linked with the amount of weight gain. Various hormonal theories have also been postulated. These include an excess of estrogen, an estrogen-progesterone imbalance, an excess of progesterone, an excess of pituitary antidiuretic hormone, and allergy to estrogen or progesterone. Some researchers feel that psychological factors are dominant, because the syndrome seems to be worse in the more neurotic. Still others feel the syndrome is predominantly a combination of hormonal factors interwoven with psychic factors.

Since premenstrual tension in its typical form occurs only in women who ovulate, anything which inhibits ovulation will also prevent the syndrome. However, this would involve month-long therapy. Instead, a good deal can be accomplished by treatment with diuretics just during the few days or even week or two of symptoms. If some symptoms still remain, progesterone is frequently added. A tranquilizer is often helpful, as is reassurance. Testosterone, the male hormone, in small doses for a week preceding ovulation, frequently does the trick alone. Its mechanism of action is obscure. Benefit is probably due to its inhibition of high estrogen build-up at this time of the cycle. As though this isn't confusing enough, some have found estrogen itself helpful in this syndrome.

Several different methods of therapy can be tried to see which helps a particular woman most. Most women can be substantially or completely relieved of this monthly annoyance by repeating the effective medication each cycle.

Just as estrogen deficiency may be undesirable, so is an *overabundance* of estrogen, which is believed in some cases to be a cause of premenstrual tension. When this is the case, an anti-estrogen often prevents the symptoms. While progesterone can do this, I've had the best results with testosterone. I give this for a few days during the week preceding ovulation, for it is then that estrogen usually builds up. Such therapy has *no* effect upon ovulation, and the dosage is small enough so there are usually no side effects. It not only helps the symptoms that would ordinarily occur with the approach of the coming menstrual period, but often makes that period much more comfortable.

Only recently I saw a young woman of 27 who had suffered with severe premenstrual symptoms for years. Diuretics had given her only moderate relief. On her first month of therapy, consisting only of small doses of testosterone for a week preceding ovulation, she reported that for the first time in years she hadn't the slightest twinge of premenstrual symptoms. And as an added bonus she was pleasantly surprised to find that her period was painless.

Another patient, an actress, was completely incapacitated by premenstrual tension. The week before her period was due, she was irritable and depressed. If she had a tragic role this worked out well, since she felt weepy anyway. She did not respond favorably to simple therapy such as diuretics or testosterone, and relief came only when ovulation was completely suppressed.

To the woman who does not want children, any delay in the arrival of the menstrual period is fraught with great tension and worry. When and if it does come, it is considered a blessing.

Quite the opposite is the reaction of the woman who hopes to become pregnant. Each slight delay is accompanied by the greatest hope and expectation, while each onset of menstruation is met with keen disappointment.

Menstruation in this country starts at about the age of thirteen or fourteen. It marks the beginning of "nubility", or womanhood. The first few menstrual periods are usually irregular and not accompanied by ovulation. When ovulation becomes cyclic, a regular menstrual pattern is established. This is the beginning of reproductive life, which lasts about thirty years. Somewhere in the mid-forties ovulation again begins to falter, and menstruation becomes irregular. Its final cessation marks the menopause and, with it, the end of being able to have a child.

The menopause signifies the end of menstruation due to a physiologic decline in ovarian hormonal function at an age which averages 49 in this country. It is not possible to "postpone" the menopause in the sense that one cannot postpone the decline of ovarian function. One may, however, postpone the cessation of menstrual periods by inducing cyclic bleeding with hormone therapy. This can be continued indefinitely if the doctor or patient wishes it. However, such therapy has no effect upon reproductive function. With or without hormonal therapy, fertility is on the wane when a woman is in her forties. Chances of pregnancy approach zero around the age of fifty, even if menstruation is still occurring naturally.

104

Menstrual periods may be heavy or light, long or short, painful or painless. During reproductive years, the presence of premenstrual tension or painful periods usually signifies a regular ovulatory pattern. Women who do not ovulate usually have painless periods with no premenstrual tension. *However, the reverse is not true.* That is, the absence of pain or tension does *not* mean that something is wrong with ovulation, which can occur quite normally and regularly in the absence of any discomfort. Moreover, painful menstruation may be associated with endometriosis (the presence of bits of uterine lining outside the womb or in the wall of the womb) and this may be associated with impaired fertility.

Menstruation is actually the *end* of a monthly cyclic process rather than the beginning. It was once thought that menstruation marked the most fertile time of a woman's cycle, corresponding to that of animals in heat. Only with the discovery that ovulation takes place about two weeks before each menstrual period was it understood that menstruation really represented a woman's most infertile time. The "rhythm" method of contraception is based on this principle, the "safe period" individually calculated as a certain number of days immediately surrounding menstruation.

Not too much attention is paid to menstruation as long as it's not too heavy, too light, or too uncomfortable —and as long as it comes "on time" when it's wanted, and fails to come when pregnancy is desired.

But it's a rare woman who goes through life without some menstrual problem at one time or another.

All women experience occasional irregularities in their menstrual cycles. In fact, it has been said that there is nothing so regular about a woman's menstrual cycle as its irregularity.

However, when a woman notes an obvious deviation

from her usual pattern, she becomes understandably concerned. It would be important and reassuring for her to know what types of vaginal bleeding are considered medically abnormal and which are of little significance. For example, an occasional heavy period need not be of concern. Neither should the presence of small clots be alarming. Clots are simply the result of more rapid flow, with insufficient time for the blood to liquify. Sometimes bleeding or spotting from the bladder or the rectum is mistaken for vaginal bleeding. A simple way of differentiating is to insert a tampon into the vagina for a day.

The following types of bleeding, however, should be considered abnormal: Repeatedly profuse or prolonged (over a week) menstrual periods, unexpected bleeding between periods, or bleeding after the menopause. There is one exception. The scant spotting many women have for a day or so during the mid-cycle (two weeks premenstrually) is due to passage of the egg (ovulation) and is not abnormal.

A woman should consult her doctor for abnormal bleeding so that he may determine the cause and give her proper therapy. Uppermost in most women's minds is the fear of cancer. Widespread newspaper and magazine publicity have helped create a cancer consciousness among all of us. This is fortunate when it prompts an early diagnosis. But it is unfortunately often the cause of unwarranted anxiety. The fact is, cancer is not the leading cause of abnormal vaginal bleeding. But since it is the most important and serious of the possible causes, it must always be considered.

For the complaint of abnormal or irregular bleeding, the physician will ask pertinent questions and will do a careful physical examination. If the bleeding has occurred after a delayed period, he will determine if it has anything to do with pregnancy. This too is always a consideration in a woman of childbearing age. If not related to pregnancy, the doctor may want to make one or more special tests, including "Pap" smears, to help determine the cause of the irregular bleeding.

The vaginal smear has become popularly known as the "cancer test". It is true that the primary purpose of such smears is to detect the presence of any abnormal-looking cells that may be cast off from the cervix or uterine cavity. Actually, the "Pap" smear is more a preventive test than a diagnostic one. It will alert the physician to look further. But it is not possible to make a conclusive diagnosis on the basis of a smear alone. Even if abnormal-looking cells are found, it does not necessarily indicate the existence of cancer, for minor infections in the genital tract can produce such a picture. By the same token, a smear reported as "negative" does not mean there is no possibility of cancer, though such a report is certainly comforting.

There are also other tests to investigate abnormal bleeding. The "biopsy" involves taking a few bits of tissue from the cervix or from the uterine cavity for more elaborate microscopic examination of areas that need further study. Then there is the hysterogram, which is an x-ray of the inside of the womb to note any irregularities in contour which may contribute to abnormal bleeding, such as polyps or fibroids. Finally, there is the "curettage"—also known as "D and C" (a dilatation of the cervix, and curettage of the uterine lining). This is a scraping of the lining of the womb for tissue examination. While this procedure is primarily done for diagnosis, it is often curative as well—for example, when bleeding is due to polyps within the womb, and are removed during the operation. Since anesthesia is needed, hospitalization is required for a day or two.

As a rule, bleeding between periods or after the menopause will require more extensive investigation than heavy, but regular periods.

Happily, the majority of cases of abnormal bleeding seen in office practice are due to a simple glandular imbalance. For this reason, such cases are termed "functional" or "dysfunctional" bleeding. This is almost always the cause when abnormal bleeding occurs in adolescent or young women. In older age groups, the diagnosis of functional bleeding cannot be made with certainty until organic causes have been eliminated.

One of the first things the doctor will want to know is whether a woman is taking any hormones for menopausal or postmenopausal symptoms. This question is no longer limited to the older age groups, since any woman taking birth control pills is in effect taking similar hormones. Regulation of dosage may be all that is needed in the case of younger women taking oral contraceptives. But the older woman on estrogen replacement therapy must be individually investigated if she has unexpected bleeding. The indiscriminate or unsupervised use of female hormones for menopausal symptoms is a frequent cause of abnormal bleeding. If stopping the pills does not cause cessation of bleeding, further investigation is required.

In the absence of pill-taking as a cause of abnormal bleeding, the treatment of bleeding due to glandular imbalance is with appropriate hormones such as estrogen, progesterone, testosterone, thyroid—according to the results of the examination and tests.

Sometimes a readily detectable cause is found on initial examination and no further tests are necessary. For example, there may be a polyp—a small, fleshy growth—in the cervix. This can be easily and painlessly removed in the office. Another common cause is an "erosion" of the cervix. This is simply a rawness due to local bacteria. Office treatment is by cautery, which is not painful due to the absence of heat nerves in this area. Still another easily detectable cause of irregular spotting which occurs in postmenopausal women is the presence of thinned-out vaginal tissues containing raw spots due to hormonal lack. This condition is also amenable to immediate treatment.

A great many women of all ages have firm, rounded overgrowths of uterine muscle and fibrous tissue in the womb called "fibroid tumors". Such tumors are not associated with cancer. They are so common that one out of three women past the age of forty has them. Most often they cause no symptoms at all, and the patient is surprised, during routine examination, to hear the doctor mention they are present.

Whether or not fibroids cause abnormal bleeding depends more upon their location than their size. Fibroids located on the outside surface of the womb are not likely to have much effect upon the menstrual period unless they are quite large. On the other hand, if a fibroid, even a small one, projects into the inner cavity of the womb, it can produce profuse bleeding. Such fibroids cannot be felt on pelvic examination, but can usually be detected by x-ray of the womb, or noted during curettage.

When fibroids are large (bigger than a three-month size pregnancy) or cause persistently troublesome bleeding despite conservative hormonal measures, the treatment is surgical. In young women, particularly those planning to have more children, an attempt is made to remove just the fibroids, leaving the main portion of the womb intact. In older women or in those who have completed their families, it is usually better to remove the entire uterus, since this also prevents the recurrence of fibroids as well as any other diseases of the uterus. Fibroids usually begin to "shrink" after the menopause, probably due to diminished hormonal output. Conversely, fibroids may be stimulated to grow faster when estrogens are administered. However, rapid growth may also occur without additional estrogen. Such rapid growth also warrants surgery.

At the approach of menopause, periods are normally scantier, and there may be either a wider interval between them or else there is complete cessation. Other patterns are considered abnormal—heavier periods, more frequent periods, or bleeding between periods. Irregular bleeding of this sort cannot simply be ascribed to the "changes".

A woman should be aware of the fact that *post-menopausal* bleeding is an entirely different matter. In the absence of hormone ingestion, any bleeding occurring one year or more after cessation of menstruation is abnormal and requires curettage to rule out a malignancy or other pathologic condition.

On the other hand, it is reassuring to note that if a woman has had no periods for several months, then has a "period" which is *preceded* by the various premenstrual symptoms and signs of old, such as backache and breast soreness, it is pretty good evidence that her ovaries have begun to put out a sizable quantity of estrogen again. This bleeding is not alarming.

11

Pleasure without Pain

We that live to please, must please to live.
SAMUEL JOHNSON

No matter what the age of the couple, the sexual relationship between husband and wife is an integral part of their total relationship. As we get older, special sexual problems of an emotional nature do arise, but there is one particular physical problem that is quite common in women after menopause. This is the gradual thinning and drying of the vaginal tissues, due to estrogen deprivation, which makes intercourse painful.

This was the problem that brought Mrs. W. to me. She was a healthy, evidently well adjusted woman of 55, whose menopause had been ten years ago. For the past two years, she experienced vaginal irritation and discomfort during intercourse with a slight staining afterwards for a few days. There was marked atrophy—that is, thinning and reddening of the entire vaginal mucosa. Simply rubbing with a swab produced staining from this area. There was also reddening externally at the entrance to the vagina. The smear, of course, showed a marked preponderance of "atrophy" (parabasal) cells and also many white (pus) cells. An estrogenic ointment was prescribed and the patient was told she could resume intercourse in about a week. When I saw her again, three weeks later, the vaginal mucosa looked quite healthy. The patient reported painless intercourse for the first time in two years. There was no further staining.

She should have come for help as soon as she had found intercourse uncomfortable. But like many women, she thought it was an unfortunate part of aging and couldn't be helped. Only when the condition began to cause bleeding did she come for medical attention. Why estrogen deficiency in some cases should single out the vaginal mucosa and produce no other symptoms is unknown.

Normally the vagina is moist, soft and elastic. The extent of its elasticity is quite amazing when one considers that this slender, tubular structure can stretch widely enough to let a baby pass through it. (The "cut" that obstetricians often make at the time of delivery is not primarily in the stretchable vagina but rather in the thick, tense muscles below it.)

With advancing years the vagina in some women begins to lose its elasticity. As estrogen deprivation becomes more severe, the vaginal lips become thin and shrunken, the vaginal lining becomes roughened and ulcerated, and an inflammatory reaction sets in which leads to itching, irritation, and either discharge or dryness. The condition is known as atrophic vaginitis.

Because of these physical changes, intercourse becomes increasingly painful. Sometimes the itching around the vulva leads a woman to seek relief in increased sexual relations. This only causes more irritation. Often a woman is quite comfortable unless sexual intercourse is attempted. This makes sex seem the culprit. The real cause is vaginal atrophy, and coitus merely aggravates the preexisting condition.

The problem is of equal concern to the husband. He is understandably dismayed that sex, formerly associated with pleasure, now brings pain. Indeed, his wife's obvious displeasure is both a physical and psychological deterrent to his sexual approaches. At the same time, the wife who develops guilt about intercourse and believes that all the difficulty is hers should bear in mind that sexual inadequacy in middle age is not exclusively a woman's problem. The *male* organ can also show signs of aging.

When I see an atrophic vaginal state and the patient has "no complaints", I know that sex relations must be at a complete standstill. Or when questions relating to sex evoke an answer such as, "I can't remember the last time," it tells the story of the physical side of that marriage. In other cases there is almost no awareness of the lack: "My husband? Oh, he's very considerate. He doesn't bother me at all."

But not all women ignore vaginal discomforts. Embarrassed to discuss such matters with a physician, many will first try home remedies such as common lubricating jellies or creams. While lubricants may ease some of the discomforts, they will not affect the basic cause of the problem—estrogen deficiency.

The diagnosis should be made by a physician. He will suspect atrophic vaginitis from the appearance of the vulvar and vaginal tissues. A drop of vaginal secretion under a microscope will reveal the typical atrophy cells, and will also serve to exclude other common causes of itching and irritation, such as fungus or trichomonas parasitic infection.

Once the diagnosis of atrophic vaginitis is made, treatment is specific. The simplest therapy is estrogen applied locally, in the form of a cream or estrogen suppositories. Estrogen by mouth may be used instead, or in addition.

Improvement is dramatically fast. Within a week or two the vaginal tissues change from a tender, thin, dry, brittle state to the normally moist, thicker, more elastic, nontender state. A drop of secretion under the microscope now reveals an entirely different picture. Gone are most—if not all—of the atrophy cells and in their place are normal vaginal lining cells. Gone too are the complaints of itching, irritation and painful intercourse.

How estrogen works on the vaginal tissues is an exciting story. Recent work indicates that estrogen plays a vital role in the life processes of at least certain cells, that is, in cell metabolism. A fascinating experiment was done by Dr. Sheldon Segal and co-workers at the Population Council Laboratories at Rockefeller University, New York. A rat that had two uteri was the subject. Estrogen was applied to one uterus but not the other. It was found that for genital organ cells (such as the uterus), certain materials essential to cellular life could be restored only by applying estrogen. Thus estrogen can stimulate target cells such as the vagina or uterus, but it can't stimulate non-target cells such as the lungs. Other body tissues and organs have not been studied sufficiently to classify into target or non-target cells.

Since the treatment of vaginal atrophy is hormonal, it should always be under medical supervision. Inasmuch as vaginal atrophy is not a temporary condition, however, the tissues will eventually revert to an atrophic state if left untreated for months or years. Therefore it is quite probable that, lacking an outside estrogen supply, a woman with this condition will require repeated hormonal nourishment, depending upon the symptoms and the physician's finding at periodic examinations. If there is ever a time when the expression "estrogen for life" can be applied, it is certainly for atrophic vaginal states.

There are two other common conditions that can cause identical symptoms of vaginal itching, irritation and painful intercourse, namely, monilia and trichomonas. A correct diagnosis is important since treatment for each one is different.

Monilia is a fungus infection. It sometimes follows the use of antibiotics, which tend to kill off normal, protective vaginal bacteria and allow uninhibited growth of fungus. But usually the exact reason for its occurrence, or recurrence, is obscure. The diagnosis is confirmed by noting the typical fungus spores on microscopic examination, or by special growth media. There are a good many different remedies

114

(various suppositories, jellies, purple dyes, douches) which may be effective. The exact medication prescribed seems to be less important than the diligence and persistence of treatment. Sometimes the intestinal tract is found to be the source of fungus, and this is treated by oral medication.

The trichomonad is a tiny parasite with several whip-like tails that enable it to move about. Due to this motion it is readily identified under the microscope. The source is unknown. Recently a new oral preparation has proven extremely effective in eradicating the condition. Recurrences are sometimes due to the husband, who can carry the infection as a "silent partner" without knowing it. Treating the husband with the same medication solves this problem.

There are still other, less common causes of vaginal itching and irritation, which your physician may have to investigate. Also, if the discharge is blood-tinged, and this is not due to local causes, other causes, including malignancy of the genital tract, must be considered.

But by far the most common cause of simple vaginal irritation in the older woman is atrophic vaginitis, which is readily reversible with estrogen. The cause is a hormonal deficiency; the lack is obvious; the treatment is specific. Both the patient and her husband are most grateful.

For to human beings, making love is very important. In fact, humans are the only species to make love at all seasons.

Porcupines, for instance, mate once a year (can you blame them?) Elephants, on the other hand, have a rather long courting season. But copulation may finally take only a minute. Some animals such as foxes and wolves remain monogamous for life. Others such as baboons maintain harems. Interestingly, those animals that most resemble the human—monkeys and chimpanzees—seem to have a stressful sex life.

A telling indictment of the human race was made recently by the naturalist Lorenz. He suggested that man may well be the missing link between apes and humans.

All human societies have always had some sort of marital relationship as part of the culture. And all have rules about it. Some of the most primitive societies such as the Manbutis of the Congo or the Semang of Malaya maintain monogamous marriages with practically no adultery. Other tribes, of course, have had polygamous customs, including the "buying" or "capturing" of women. The ancient Greeks had a rather contemptuous regard for marriage and women. They felt that wives should be seen but not heard. Roman women had a lot more freedom. But emancipation came slowly. As late as the mid-nineteenth century, an American wife could not own property or even have legal control of her own children.

In other times marriages were prearranged. Now they are made presumably for "love". According to one psychiatrist, this practically guarantees future problems because the choosing of a mate is one of the most ill-prepared-for and confused steps a person takes, "not primarily because he (or she) chooses a mate whose interests and habits are incompatible with his own, but because each of the pair is ignorant of the unconscious purposes that determine their respective choices".

In spite of such handicaps, 75 percent of American marriages have somehow stumbled into middle age. Someone has said that the sex life of the older person is almost as poorly understood as the sex life of teenagers but the reasons are different. In the case of teenagers, they won't talk. In the case of older people, nobody asks.

I disagree with the claim that sex is "better than ever" when a woman reaches menopause because she's free from the fear of pregnancy and for the first time in her life can be spontaneous. In this day of sophisticated contraception, the onset of menopause hardly makes a difference. And I've met few women who were pleased that their reproductive function was over, even though they did not expect to use it. As far as sexual spontaneity is concerned, if they have never been spontaneous before, chances are the menopause will not make them so.

It's true that sometimes a flurry of sexual activity accompanies the onset of the menopause. This is not due to a sudden interest in sex itself—but, rather, a feeling that the gates of reproduction are about to close. In the last century, a medical article on menopause had a similar suggestion: ". . . there is a sudden increase in sexual desire, which, at the change of life, may be compared to the last waking up of a soon to be extinguished flame. . . ."

This fear has persisted. And many women today still equate the end of menstruation with the end of pleasurable sex life. They feel that a decline in sex hormones means a decline in libido.

Like so many other menopausal symptoms, this decline in libido, if it does occur, is not the direct result of diminished hormonal production. It is related to other problems of middle age.

What, then, is the relationship of sex homones to sex drive in the average woman? First, one cannot directly increase or decrease the sex drive of a woman of any age by giving her estrogen, the chief female sex homone. This is true whether she is estrogen-deficient or not.

Second, erotic goals are not dependent on the presence of hormones, but are culturally determined. This was clearly demonstrated in an interesting study of children suffering from precocious puberty. Despite their *ability* to respond as adults because of their maturation, their erotic goals were appropriate for their chronological age.

Third, surgical removal of the ovaries of women even below the age of forty does not interfere with their sexual desires.

Fourth, if estrogen production were alone responsible

117

for a woman's sexual capacity, one would expect a fairly uniform decline in response among women as they got older. We know that there is no such correlation.

Fifth, detailed case histories of many women of middle age have shown continual sexual responsiveness as compared with earlier years.

But the menopause, the decline in hormonal production, the middle years, all may have an *indirect* influence, both physically and psychologically, on a woman's sexual capacity and drive. Certain physical changes of estrogen deprivation may interfere with sex, such as thinning of the vaginal mucous membrane. Many women with vaginal atrophy complain of discomfort *only* with intercourse. The association of sex with pain becomes an obvious deterrent to any satisfactory sexual relationship. Some also have pain on urination following intercourse, due to similar thinning of the urethral and bladder lining. Since this lining is located right next to the vagina, it is easy to see how sexual activity can irritate both areas at once. The important point is that in 85 percent of cases where *painful* intercourse is the complaint, the cause is physical rather than psychological.

Other physiological results of estrogen deprivation, such as flushes, night sweats, insomnia and fatigue, may indirectly interfere with sexual responsiveness. Alleviating the various discomforts of the menopause will help such women enjoy the physical relationship at least to the same degree as before menopause.

Another cause of sexual difficulty peculiar to the older woman is relaxation of the vaginal tissues. Although previous childbirth may have started the weakening process, the combination of years of pelvic pressure, thinning of the fibromuscular supports, and estrogen decline all contribute to the relaxed state. As far as sex is concerned, there may be too little friction for male satisfaction. Some cases respond to special vaginal exercises; others require surgical correction.

In short, if a woman is in good health, feels well, *and has always had a good sex life*, there is no reason to expect any sudden change because of the menopause. Masters and Johnson studied the sex responses of a select group of postmenopausal women, and reported that clitoral response continues into the seventy-year age group in patterns not unlike premenopausal women. They also found that orgasm was unchanged, except for being of shorter duration than in younger women, sometimes accompanied by painful uterine contractions. There was also less vaginal lubrication in older women. The few exceptions were women who had maintained an active sex life. The authors concluded that the older woman needs an even more regular sex life than the younger one, to maintain proper lubrication and vaginal distensibility.

The postmenopausal woman does need a regular sex life. But nature has slipped up somewhere, because it is likely that her husband, who is probably older, has a simultaneous diminution of needs, if not of potency, which becomes particularly apparent in his sixties and seventies. Unless a woman is aware of this she may believe herself rejected.

Someone has plotted a graph showing two lines. The first represents male libido. It starts high, since the male sex drive is supposed to be highest around age 18 or 19, and slowly, gradually declines. The wife's graph of sexual capacity starts relatively low and, in a typical female pattern, gradually rises with advancing years. Somewhere in the middle, around age 32, the two graphs meet—for about an hour!

But not all women have increased sexual urges as they get older. Many, in fact, experience just the opposite. But the alteration of responsiveness is psychological. Many women use the excuse of the "changes" or of advancing years to avoid sexual relations. Chances are they were never really interested anyway.

Sex is more a matter of the mind and heart than of the genital organs.

Nevertheless, when a woman feels that her desire or response is not all it should be, she often asks if there is any hormone that might improve her libido. Oddly enough, estrogen, the female sex hormone, will neither increase nor decrease the sex drive in the human female (though it will in animals). But the male hormone, testosterone, will frequently increase the sex desires of those women who previously had a good response. The results may be quite successful, but much depends on the husband's reaction. Some men say, "Whatever it is you're giving her, don't stop."

Others cry, "Help!"

But there is no corresponding drug that will help male libido. Giving estrogen to men will generally diminish both their desire and potency. In fact, hormonal therapy of any kind is likely to fail.

Occasionally it is desirable to *decrease* female libido, for example in an elderly woman who is bothered by erotic dreams. The use of the hormone progesterone will usually accomplish this.

Some patients complain of feeling "oversexed". One that comes to mind was a single woman, Miss W. She was 49, and had her last menstrual period a half year ago. She was considerably bothered by heightened libido. Except for a low estrogen activity on the smear, she was in good physical shape. But estrogen therapy didn't help her. It was progesterone that succeeded in alleviating what she considered her oversexed emotions. Just as testosterone is the drug which can frequently heighten a woman's libido, progesterone is the one that can have the most effect in lessening such feelings. Usually rather high doses are necessary.

Another patient, this one with a poor libido, was given a different estrogen preparation, one which contained a fair amount of the male hormone, testosterone, specifically to stimulate the libido. Mrs. E. had had a hysterectomy two years ago and it had seemed to her that recently her response to sex had been poor and her desire equally sluggish. Two months later, I asked whether the treatment had any effect. "A little too good at times," she said.

Increased libido in the female has also been reported after the application of local vaginal cream containing testosterone, the cream having been given for some other condition.

Incidentally, the increased sex drive that results from testosterone administration does not mean that the woman was deficient in that hormone. There are instances where one benefits from the pharmacological action of a drug without being deficient in it. For example, giving adrenaline helps asthma, even though there is no deficiency of adrenaline.

Aphrodisiacs have been effective mainly in folklore. The ancient Greeks believed that certain foods had magical powers which enhanced the sex drive—particularly onions and garlic, because these root vegetables have the shape of male testicles.

The older woman has always had her special problems. In the last century she didn't dare express sexual feelings. "Excessive sexual desire at the menopause is indicative of disease," wrote one doctor in 1894. A generation ago, husbands complained that their wives were unresponsive. Now wives complain that their husbands don't satisfy them. Sex, being fraught with tension, guilt and anxiety, is often given as the reason for divorce.

Sometimes it is not until later years that a woman finds herself suddenly confronted by a serious marital problem. Children are away from home; husband and wife are quite alone with each other. If they have not communicated well before, the process of aging may make matters worse. Even illness, which is more common in the elderly, can aggravate marriage problems, and many family practitioners involuntarily find themselves in the role of counselors.

Of interest is the question of how much lack of communication and interest is due to the husband's diminishing desires. Is there a "male menopause"?

Men, of course, have no menopause, that is, cessation of the menses. But some men go through a transitional change. This is not a result of any hormonal deficiency. The main change involves their thinking habits—worrying about unfulfilled ambitions, wondering about a waning sex drive, and worrying about their menopausal wives. Such emotional changes are no more pathological than similar emotional changes in the female. The forties and fifties are a time of readjustment for everyone.

(Even doctors are not immune. Prompted by a concern for what was aptly termed "the intellectual menopause", an editorial in a medical journal deplored the fact that some doctors drop out of the world of medicine to escape the pressures of their profession, and urged that the age of maturity is the wrong time to quit.)

Men must pass through middle age too. True, there is no end of menstruation to mark the time. And more important, there is no sudden hormonal shift—androgen levels decline very slowly. Nor does reproductive function end, as it does for women, at middle age. In fact, men can reproduce far into old age. There are reliable reports of men becoming fathers in their seventies, eighties and even ninties!

Although the female stops producing ova at the menopause or before, there is no sudden change in the rate of sperm manufacture in men as they get older. Sperm studies of young and middle-aged men have shown that there is no correlation between any aspect of semen analysis and man's age. As the man passes from middle to old age, there may be some decrease in sperm production, but apparently not enough to interfere with fertility. Sperm motility remains undiminished in old age as long as the frequency of intercourse is not markedly reduced. But the most interesting aspect of sperm is the morphology—the various structural shapes seen on stained smear. So constant is this that some men may be identified by their sperm, as though they were fingerprints.

Just as a woman's libido is not dependent on her estrogen output, any loss of sex drive or potency in the aging male is not the result of diminished hormonal secretion. In both the male and female, changes in libido are due more to cerebral factors than to genital ones.

Many men, in fact, maintain a strong and steady sex drive throughout life. If diminished potency occurs at all, it is probably due to a change in a man's emotional reaction to erotic stimuli, or a lack of such stimuli. Kinsey reported that about three-fourths of the men in his sample were still potent at seventy, and one-fourth at eighty.

It is perhaps fortunate that men do not undergo a true menopause. One per household is plenty. But men don't want to grow old either. Men, too, have difficulty with the "middle-age spread". Men, too, develop skin wrinkles, farsightedness, and other signs of aging.

But the most common aging feature in men is the tendency to baldness. One often hears it said that baldness in men signifies increased virility. The late Sir Cedric Hardwicke, himself sparse of hair, put it this way: "Baldness may indicate masculinity, but it diminishes one's opportunity to find out."

Medical science remains as baffled by male baldness as by the common cold. The problem is an ancient one; the cause usually hereditary. Early Egyptian prescriptions included a mixture of equal parts of hippopotamus, crocodile, lion, serpent and goose. Another consisted of a compound of dog toes, horse's hooves and date refuse. None has solved the problem. Not even catchy ads such as "At last! A Sure Cure for Baldness"—which advertises men's hair-pieces. One out of three men suffers from premature baldness.

While the male sex hormone, testosterone, is the key to body and scalp hair, most cases of male baldness are due to hereditary factors. Hereditary baldness never develops in those who fail to reach sexual maturity. That is, if a boy is castrated before puberty, he does not become bald. The adult eunuch is beardless, but seldom bald. If he is given testosterone his beard will begin to grow, and he will start losing his scalp hair if so predisposed by heredity.

Which reminds me of Don Herold's succinct comment on baldness: "Anyway, it's neat."

12

When Surgery Is Needed

When carving my middle
Be sure you don't fiddle
With matters that do not concernya
HEYWOOD BROUN

Surgery is more frequent in middle age. The older one gets, the more chance there is of something going askew.

In women, the breasts and genital organs are especially prone to disorders after forty. Understandably, a woman feels that surgery on her female organs threatens her femininity. In fact, *any* pelvic operation is likely to produce a good deal of anxiety. She wonders if the surgery will make her any less a woman, whether it will make her less attractive or change her sexual appetite or response. The answer is no. Such surgery will *not* cause these changes.

By far the most common pelvic operation is a "hysterectomy", the removal of the uterus. When the entire uterus, including the cervix, is removed, it is called a "total" or "complete" hysterectomy. If the cervix is left in, it is called a "subtotal" or "supracervical" or "partial" hysterectomy. If the uterus is removed "from below" (vaginally), it is called a "vaginal hysterectomy".

There are many reasons for a hysterectomy. The most common is enlarging or troublesome fibroids. The majority of fibroids can be left alone, particularly since they tend to

125

shrink after menopause. Sometimes even moderately large fibroids can just be "watched" from year to year, when it is more important for the patient's welfare to avoid an operation. I have in mind a 47-year-old woman who first came to me sixteen years ago at the age of 31. She had moderately large fibroids, but was unmarried and reluctant to have any kind of pelvic operation. She was in analysis, and her analyst felt such an operation would be emotionally devastating. Fortunately, her fibroids did not produce menstrual irregularities or hemorrhages and so no treatment was necessary other than observation at regular intervals. The fibroids did enlarge somewhat over the next decade, but not to alarming proportions. For the past three years, since the onset of her menopause, they have decreased in size.

Not all fibroids are so cooperative. Those which project into the cavity of the womb (submucous fibroids) have a nasty habit of causing uncontrollable bleeding episodes, not responding even to potent hormonal therapy. I recall one such patient, Miss L., a woman in her forties, whose examination disclosed only small fibroids on the surface of her womb. However, an x-ray of the inside of her womb revealed a submucous fibroid the size of a golf ball, which explained her hemorrhages. Hysterectomy was the only way to solve her problem.

Hysterectomy is also indicated when sheer size of fibroids is enough to cause pressure on surrounding structures, even if there are no bleeding problems.

In younger women who want to have children, it is often possible to remove the fibroids while leaving the main portion of the uterus intact. Mrs. J., age 31, had one child, then two miscarriages. Examination disclosed fairly large fibroids, which were removed, leaving the body of the uterus intact. She has had two normal children since. There has been a slight regrowth of her fibroids, but not enough to require any further surgical intervention.

Fortunately, fibroids hardly ever become malignant. However, hysterectomy is usually indicated if there are persistent atypical features in the lining of the uterus, or recurrent abnormal bleeding despite conservative therapy (with or without fibroids). And, of course, a proven cancer of the uterine lining is always an indication for surgery.

Some cases of uterine prolapse (descent) are also managed by hysterectomy via the vaginal route, even if the uterus is structurally normal.

Contrary to popular belief, hysterectomy alone does not produce a sudden "change of life". The latter, along with some of its disagreeable symptoms, is controlled by the ovaries, and as long as even one of the ovaries (or a portion of it) is left intact, the actual "change of life" will occur whenever ovarian function would normally diminish for that particular woman.

The term used for removal of the ovaries is "oophorectomy" or "ovariectomy". Whenever a woman undergoes a hysterectomy, there's always the question of whether the ovaries should be left in (to prevent surgical menopause) or taken out (to prevent future ovarian disease, either benign or malignant). If the ovaries had no function after middle age, the question would be academic. They would be routinely removed. However, we know that the ovaries may produce appreciable quantities of estrogen for years after the menopause. In fact, hot flushes can appear in a woman whose ovaries are removed, even if her menopause occurred years before the operation.

Removing normal looking ovaries thus may be questionable at any age, but especially in younger women. One authoritative report noted that not more than 15 percent of women are likely to be subjected to abdominal operation after the age of forty. If all ovaries were removed in this entire group, the eventual incidence of ovarian cancer would be reduced only from 8 to 7 cases in each 1,000 operated on. Many surgeons agree that leaving one or both ovaries bring advantages that far outweigh the potential risk involved. In fact, the risk of ovarian malignancy appears to be actually less in patients who have had a hysterectomy than in the general female population. Nevertheless, it is a decision for the individual surgeon to make. Some draw the line at a certain age, such as fifty, and remove ovaries after that time. Others may have a policy of not removing any normal ovaries. Then one or two previously operated patients return a few years later with cancer of the ovary, and they begin to remove ovaries "prophylactically" again.

Of course, sometimes one or both ovaries must be removed for definite pathology. If only one is removed, the other takes over the function for both. However, if both are removed while a woman is still in her reproductive years, so-called "surgical menopause" takes place, and menstruation ceases. That's why, if both ovaries must be removed, the uterus is usually removed as well, since it becomes useless and subject to possible future disorders.

Although the effects of surgical menopause are usually more severe than natural menopause, it is easy enough to give immediate estrogen replacement. Nor can such patients have any vaginal bleeding problems as a result of hormonal therapy, since the womb is absent.

How premenopausal patients feel after surgery often depends on whether or not the ovaries have been removed.

Mrs. F. is now 53. I removed her uterus twelve years ago because of troublesome fibroids, leaving the ovaries in. She has felt well since the operation and the only complaint has been some recent vaginal irritation which cleared up with the use of local estrogen.

In contrast, Mrs. N. is now 54. I removed her uterus *and ovaries* fourteen years ago because of large ovarian cysts and fibroids. She needed estrogen therapy within a few days of her operation and has required fairly high doses ever since. If she stops the pills or even decreases the dosage, flushes and sweats recur.

When a relatively young woman's ovaries are removed, she will usually feel much better if estrogen replacement is started early (provided there are no contraindications). I use estrogen by injection postoperatively, switching to oral medication in a few days when the patient is able to tolerate drugs by mouth. It is rarely necessary to use estrogen by injection, but this is one of the exceptions.

Whether the symptoms that follow surgical removal of the ovaries are due directly to the suppression of ovarian function or to the emotional effects of such suppression, it's important that women realize that such operations will not make them any less attractive or less responsive sexually.

As a woman advances in age, a frequent complaint is a progressive relaxation of the pelvic supports resulting in a "bulge" noticeable at the vaginal entrance. When the bulge is mainly a herniation of the uterus itself, it is known as uterine "prolapse". When it is mainly the vaginal tissue overlying the bladder, it is called a "cystocele". When it involves the rectal wall, it is termed "rectocele". All three may occur together. Such relaxations are sometimes accompanied by bladder symptoms such as involuntary loss of urine, or urinary urgency.

Previous childbirth may weaken the pelvic supports initially, but thinning of the tissues from loss of muscle tone and connective tissue support aggravates the process in later years. How much of this relaxation is due to estrogen deficiency and how much is due to aging alone is not known. However, the same type of relaxation may be seen in many younger, still menstruating women with no estrogen lack. But when a vaginal bulge is associated with thin, atrophic tissues, it is always helpful to use local estrogen applications. Such treatment is also helpful to assist healing after surgery.

An actual bulge of the vaginal tissues, be it herniation of the uterus, bladder or rectum, is often uncomfortable enough for a woman to seek medical help. Such a condition requires either support with a pessary or, for permanent relief, surgical correction. However, I have treated some women who complained of a "feeling of bulging", where no actual bulge existed. The feeling apparently was created by an atrophic condition of the vaginal tissues, and the sensation of a "bulge" disappeared when the thin, dry tissues were restored to normal with local estrogen therapy alone.

On the other hand, when true pelvic relaxation exists and surgical correction is chosen, one of several types of plastic repairs usually serves to tighten the loose, and bulging structures.

The repair should be good enough for the relief of symptoms. However, it must also take into account the husband. He also may be showing the effects of tissue relaxation! Therefore, vaginal plastic procedures for cosmetic reasons alone are best avoided since they may lead only to frustration for the husband. "Nature has been wise; as the turgor of the phallus decreases, the commodiousness of the vagina increases. Man would be wise to leave well enough alone, at least until he is able to repair the shaft too."

There is something about preservation of structure and function of the sexual organs that is very special and tied to the emotions. Many years ago, when I was an intern, an elderly gentleman on the ward was getting his first sponge bath by a nurse. After washing him almost everywhere, she handed him the wash cloth, saying, "Now this is for the rest of you." "Ah!" he sighed, "what was once the best of me is now the rest of me!"

Regarding vaginal relaxations in women, there is one associated condition that is always intolerable, the involuntary loss of urine. The condition is still not well understood. Apparently, different mechanisms are responsible in different patients. For this reason the operative procedure chosen must be individualized. Sometimes the use of special muscle-strengthening exercises will alleviate or even cure the condition. This is often tried prior to surgery.

Sometimes the pelvic supports give way completely, resulting in an extreme form of prolapse where the woman actually notes her womb hanging between her legs. This condition is known as "complete prolapse". It usually affects people in the 70's or even 80's. Because of senility and commonly associated medical conditions such as hypertension, cardiac disease, nephritis or diabetes, such women are poorer risks for major or prolonged surgery. Fortunately, there is a relatively simple surgical procedure which entails minimal risk and complications, consisting of "inverting" the herniation so as to close the vagina almost completely. Because of the nature of the operation, it can only be performed on those who have permanently relinquished sexual activity. If this is not the case, a modification of the procedure may be done which permits partial coitus.

Mrs. B. came to me with just such a condition. When I asked her age, she said "79 plus!" She was a spry and energetic widow, apparently in her early 80's. She had moderate vaginal bulging for years, but for the past few weeks, everything, she said, was hanging out. Examination revealed a complete herniation of the uterus, which could be replaced. However, any exertion, even ordinary walking, caused it to come out again. Moreover, the vaginal tissues were very thin and atrophic.

The vaginal tissues were first gotten into shape for surgery by local estrogen cream. The uterus was kept in place with special tampons during this therapy. Also during this interval, there was an opportunity to have her heart thoroughly checked. When cleared for surgery by her internist, a "Le Fort" operation was done, which closed off the vagina. She took the procedure well, and was out of bed on the first postoperative day. To date, she has had no re-currence of the herniation or any other complaints referable to that area. It had been explained beforehand, of course, that the operation would preclude any future coitus.

As far as surgery in old age is concerned, even some 75 years ago it was deemed advisable to operate in order to re-lieve symptoms. The following is quoted from the *Journal of the American Medical Association,* 1891:

> With regard to advanced age being a contraindi-cation to surgical operation, it is held that if a patient be in fair general health, with an heredi-tary tendency to long life, mere old age is not a reason for withholding treatment, either with a view of prolonging life, or for the relief of acute suffering.

This is even truer today with modern medical ad-vances. Gynecologists are now seeing increasing numbers of older women requiring surgical intervention for the relief of symptoms formerly accepted as "woman's lot" and part of aging. That is, older women need not accept such condi-tions as urinary incontinence or relaxation of the vagina as part of the aging process, nor need they feel that the risks of surgery are great, even at advanced age. With special precautions such as early hospital admission and careful evaluation of cardiac reserve and kidney function, major gynecological surgery can safely be performed on most eld-erly patients.

෧

13

Prevention Is Best

He that won't be counselled can't be helped.
BENJAMIN FRANKLIN

Papanicolaou's classic work on vaginal smears led to the worldwide acceptance of the "Pap" test for cancer. Actually, this test is not a final diagnosis of cancer, but indicates which cases are suspicious enough to warrant further investigation which *can* provide a definite diagnosis.

Fortunately, cancer does not "strike". It creeps up very slowly and silently, often for many years, before making an obvious appearance. That is why the "Pap" smear frequently can detect abnormal cells while they are still in their precancerous stage.

Smears from the cervix itself are valuable for the detection of early cancer of the cervix, particularly if combined with biopsies in suspicious cases. But while such smears are excellent for screening early cervical cancer, they can miss in a high percentage of cancers of the uterine body. That is why smears from the vagina are usually taken as well. Some even take smears directly from the inside of the uterine cavity by suction. Any smear of uterine cells reported as "positive" or "suspicious" must always be confirmed by curettage.

The present status of cytology for cervical cancer has been well summarized by Koss. He points out that most problems pertaining to cervical cancer could be solved if only all women over twenty could have the benefit of a correctly obtained and interpreted cervical smear. He has

133

recently recommended that the Health Department in New York make the cervical smear mandatory for every patient seeking prenatal care, just as the blood test for syphilis is compulsory.

Attempts at automatic, computerized identification of cellular abnormalities have so far been unsuccessful, but investigative work is in progress.

From the point of view of preventive medicine, every woman should have a pelvic examination annually, or twice a year if she is over forty. At this examination, the location, size, shape and consistency of the uterus and ovaries are palpated. (Normal tubes usually cannot be felt.) The cervix is then inspected for evidence of erosion, that is for superficial rawness due to local bacteria, for polyp, or other abnormalities.

Once a year, "Pap" smears for the prevention and detection of cancer are taken from the cervix, and also from the vaginal pool or uterine cavity. They may, of course, be repeated sooner should there be any abnormal symptoms or findings to warrant it. In fact, if there is persistent abnormal bleeding, cancer must be looked for by more specific methods than the "Pap" smear. A "negative" smear does not necessarily mean that cancer does not exist, and a "positive" one always needs confirmation. Bleeding between menstrual periods usually calls for a diagnostic curettage. As with most other parts of the body, the earlier cancer of the uterine lining or cervix is detected the better the prognosis. Any bleeding a year or more after the menopause is associated with malignancy frequently enough to warrant every available diagnostic measure, including curettage of the uterine lining, cervical canal and cervical biopsies.

Cancer of the ovary has its highest incidence in women between the ages of 55 and 65. Unfortunately, it is not as amenable to early detection as cancer of the uterus. On rare occasion, a "Pap" smear will show a few suspicious cells, but this test is not generally useful in cases of ovarian malignancy. The best means of detection is periodic pelvic examination with follow-up and exploration of any significant ovarian enlargement. This is the chief reason why older women should have a pelvic examination more often than once a year, even though the Pap smear is just taken annually.

There are many different pathologic types of ovarian malignancy, some more malignant than others. Treatment is by surgical removal, often followed by chemotherapy to suppress further growth activity and to prolong life.

Cancer of the breast is the most common form of cancer in women. One in eighteen women will develop the disease. About 63,000 new cases are estimated this year, with about 27,000 deaths expected. It is by far the leading cause of cancer deaths in women.

The incidence of breast cancer rises steadily with age. *Statistically,* women who have borne children and those who have nursed have a somewhat decreased incidence of breast cancer, whereas women with previous chronic breast disease or a familial history of breast cancer have a definitely higher incidence. Cultural or geographic factors apparently play a role too. Japanese women have a relatively low incidence of breast cancer, and it is practically unheard of among the Eskimos.

Self-examination of the breasts has been highly publicized in a film prepared by the American Cancer Society. Since the vast majority of breast cancers are detected by women themselves, one can appreciate the extreme importance of this procedure.

You should lie on your back and bring your left hand across the chest wall. With the flat of the fingers the entire right breast is palpated, area by area. With the arm now raised, the armpit is also palpated. The procedure is repeated on the other side, using the opposite hand.

Since the procedure is often fraught with tension, especially the first time, you should ask your doctor to point out areas of normal thickening to avoid being frightened unnecessarily.

Another helpful procedure is to sit in front of a mirror and raise your arms, to see if there are any areas of dimpling or puckering of the skin of the breasts. In those women who are still having menstrual periods, breast self-examination should be done every month as the menstrual period is waning or just over, since there is least engorgement at this time. For post-menopausal women, there should be a regular habit of checking once a month. It is entirely inadequate for a woman to wait six to twelve months until her regular visit to the doctor before breast examination.

Self-examination is important. You can become quite familiar with the "feel" of your breasts after a few such examinations. You can then pick out areas that seem nodular or at least "different" from previous examinations, and call it to your doctor's attention. It should be emphasized that the feeling of a "lump" does not in itself mean cancer. There are many benign cystic or fibrous conditions too.

Mammography, or visualization of the breasts by special x-ray technique, is now a well established diagnostic tool for the detection of breast lesions. However, it has its limitations, since about 20 percent of all breast cancers will not be demonstrated by this examination, and about 10 percent of benign breast tumors may be overread as cancer. The detection of localized cancers by mammography is more difficult in women under age 45. Both breasts should be x-rayed since about three percent of breast cancers seen by the physician are bilateral. Follow-up x-rays are useful in indistinct cases to detect subtle changes which may be clinically missed.

Several knotty problems have been posed by mammography. One is that it's difficult to define a "normal" breast—that is, to decide what proportion of fatty or glandular elements is normal in women at various ages.

Also, many more trained radiologists are needed to interpret the examinations.

Nevertheless, with a diagnostic accuracy of about 80 percent (higher when combined with clinical findings), mammography is useful whenever there is a questionable mass, fibrocystic disease, a multinodular breast, skin or nipple changes, women with large breasts difficult to palpate, or even those with cancerophobia. There are no contraindications.

At present a study is under way to determine the value of periodic screening by mammography combined with clinical examination in reducing breast cancer mortality. It should be emphasized that the result of mammography does not replace the clinical necessity for biopsy of suspected breast lesions.

Detecting breast cancer by taking a smear is limited to cases with a discharge from the nipple. As with uterine cancer, it is significant if tumor cells are seen. But if not, the possibility of cancer is not ruled out. The same is true of cells obtained from fluid aspirated from breast cysts. In short, cytology is not a substitute for standard biopsy of suspected breast lesions.

Breast thermography records skin temperature by means of a "heat" photograph. The object is to detect skin temperature elevations over inflammatory or malignant lesions. It's limited, though, since skin temperature elevations are found not only in malignancies but in some normal breasts, some benign tumors, women taking various hormones, and women more than six weeks pregnant. At present, thermography is still in the investigative stage.

Another area being investigated is the possible relation of hormones to heart disease.

The heart is a remarkable organ. No larger than a fist, it weighs only half a pound. It beats over 4,000 times an hour and pumps five quarts of blood through countless miles of your circulatory system. During strenuous activity it may pump as much as ten quarts a minute.

It begins to throb when the human embryo is only a few weeks old. In an average lifetime it beats about two and one-half *billion* times with no rest, except between beats!

The Egyptians considered the heart immortal, always embalming it separately. In fact, the heart has always fascinated mankind. Plato considered it the seat of the human soul. The heart has served poets well, as a subject and symbol of love and warmth, and the tradition is carried on in the exchange of heart-shaped cards on St. Valentine's Day.

The heart is nourished by two coronary arteries and their branches. Normally these are pliable, with a smooth lining. In abnormal states they may be thickened or have a rough, "rusty" lining (atherosclerosis). If these vessels which supply the heart with oxygenated blood become narrowed or obstructed, the condition is known as coronary heart disease. There are other types—rheumatic heart disease, which scars the valves; hypertensive heart disease which imposes an increased load; and congenital heart disease from some inborn error in development. Heart disease is also related to overweight, diabetes, thyroid disease, smoking, tension associated with high blood pressure and some infectious diseases.

Back in 1850 the average life span of women was only about two to three years more than that of men. This statistical difference has slowly widened, and the expanding gap is now considerable, leaving about 10 million widows in the United States today. Why do women live longer? Are their worries less than men's? Is it that they smoke less? Is it because a woman cries, while a man fights? Is it hormones?

One factor is certainly heart disease.

The heart ages along with all other organs. Aging of the heart begins as early as the twenties and continues steadily and progressively. However, the aging of a normal heart has been aptly compared with the ocular mechanism: "Just as distant vision is well maintained while ability to adjust for close vision is lost, so the aging heart maintains its ability to deal with its usual daily burden, while progressively losing ability to adapt to sudden increase in rate, in venous return, or in arterial resistance . . . only manifest when an unusual strain is imposed."

One of the most interesting features about coronary heart disease is the different incidence in men and women. Many surveys have pointed out that men in their thirties and forties develop the disease much more frequently than women, but in the fifties the gap narrows and after sixty the ratio is almost equal. The incidence of coronary disease in women apparently increases after menopause.

This has naturally aroused a good deal of speculation as to why women are so much more "protected" against coronary disease until advanced years. More specifically, is it their drop-off in estrogen production that causes women to lose their protection? Some studies suggest that women who have had their ovaries removed have a higher incidence of atherosclerosis and cardiac abnormalities than those whose ovaries are intact. However, other studies fail to show a difference between such groups.

If estrogens do protect against coronary heart disease, what would happen if they were given to men with coronary histories? Would they be spared more attacks? There have been several studies dealing with male patients who have had at least one coronary attack to see if administration of estrogen lowered the incidence of subsequent attacks. The results, at best, are equivocal. One study, which used enough estrogen to reduce supposedly harmful components of blood fats, revealed no difference between the treated male patients and the controls.

In another study, however, there was a definite improvement in the survival rate of the estrogen-treated men.

But this study, interestingly and surprisingly, used much smaller doses, insufficient to change that portion of the blood fats considered possibly harmful.

Still another study of middle-aged men with a history of coronary disease began with large doses of an estrogen product. Surprisingly, patients started on this high dosage within three months of their most recent coronary attack had a much higher rate of recurrence than patients given a placebo. When this disquieting group was excluded, however, the death rate for the remainder of the series was 50 percent less than for patients receiving the placebo.

The divergent results of these and other studies do not permit drawing any firm conclusions. Furthermore, some of the studies, while showing that males under estrogen treatment are offered some protection compared to groups not receiving such treatment, do not take into account the high dropout rate due to undesirable side effects of estrogen therapy in males. These include diminished libido, impotence, breast enlargement and tenderness, migraine and occasional bloating.

True, estrogens *can* change certain fatty components of the blood. But the exact significance of this in the prevention of coronary disease is uncertain.

In short, the evidence relating estrogens to coronary disease rests primarily on the fact that premenopausal women have a lower incidence of coronaries than men of comparable age. Also women whose ovaries have been removed have in some studies (not in others) a higher incidence of coronaries than those whose ovaries are intact.

But statistics are open to question. In a recent report, Furman found no clear evidence from mortality data that diminished ovarian function per se makes a woman more vulnerable to coronary disease. He believes that the higher coronary death rate in older women "approaches" the male rate not because of some sudden loss of protection, but rather because of a decreased *male* death rate, probably due to loss of large numbers of relatively young, male heart attack victims. Cultural, racial and economic factors may also play a role. For example, the American Negro woman is almost as susceptible as the male. The female/male coronary death rates are also close to each other in some less affluent countries such as Italy and Japan.

There is no evidence at present that women on estrogen replacement therapy will continue in advanced years to have the same "protection" that they enjoyed in pre-menopausal years. Hopefully, large-scale, controlled studies will show such benefit. At present there is only the negative data—that women without benefit of estrogen replacement *will* have a rising incidence of coronary disease with advancing years.

Most of the research work so far has been on men. Now, though, there are two long-range studies of *women* under way at one of the hospitals in Massachusetts. One will try to answer the question: Can estrogen delay or prevent atherosclerosis following the menopause? The other concerns women who have had coronary attacks, and will examine the value of estrogen in preventing complications of the disease and in prolonging life. It will take ten to fifteen years before definitive answers can be given.

The evidence at hand is that although estrogens may not be warranted for all women, they might be seriously considered for "high risk" coronary candidates—women in their forties with mounting blood pressure, high cholesterol, obesity, impaired thyroid function, a family history of diabetes or coronary disease, and heavy smokers.

Now let's consider cholesterol—an essential and vital part of every cell, particularly the cell membrane. It is the cholesterol in the outer layer of the skin that makes the skin "waterproof".

Cholesterol is commonly thought of as fat. Actually

it isn't a true fat but rather a steroid, related chemically to the sex steroids.

Cholesterol is found in animal protein such as meat, eggs and milk. However, the body produces its *own* cholesterol from the metabolism of carbohydrates, fats and proteins. Therefore, even if one avoided foods high in cholesterol content, one would have enough from the body's own production. Even the wall of human arteries can synthesize cholesterol, which explains why fatty plaques may be found in people with normal or even low blood cholesterol.

There is a tendency for the cholesterol level to rise with advancing age. A higher level is also associated with decreased thyroid function, diabetes, poor kidney function, the kind of animal protein eaten (e.g., eggs more than meat), diet high in saturated fatty acids, and even situations of stress.

Blood cholesterol, however, does not exist as a separate entity. It's bound to protein, such as the fatty protein component of the blood, which is found to be elevated in many coronary cases, and in many postmenopausal women. This *chemical* abnormality can be reversed in some cases with estrogen therapy. But while such treatment will change the chemical abnormality, the effect upon coronary disease and atherosclerosis is still uncertain.

The evidence linking cholesterol with rusty arteries (atherosclerosis) is also largely circumstantial. It hasn't been proven that atherosclerosis is caused by cholesterol in the diet, or that a low-fat diet prevents heart attacks. So despite a long known association between high blood cholesterol and coronary heart disease, there need not be any cause-and-effect relationship. Hopefully, a new drug that is said to lower blood cholesterol levels may shed further light on this complex subject.

Much remains to be learned. Aside from diet, we need to know a lot more about the relationship of atherosclerosis and coronary heart disease to age, heredity, race, hypertension, obesity, diabetes, occupational stress, alcohol, smoking and prolonged inactivity. A case can be made linking any one of these factors to coronary disease.

To drive home this point, the moderator of a medical symposium on atherosclerosis summed up the conclusions of the speakers by giving a composite answer to the question "What type of person is least likely to get atherosclerosis?" "The person least likely to get atherosclerosis is a hypotensive, bicycling, unemployed, hypo-beta-lipoproteinic, hyper-alpha-lipoproteinic, non-smoking, hypolipemic, underweight, premenopausal female dwarf living in a crowded room on the island of Crete before 1925 and subsisting on a diet of uncoated cereals, safflower oil and water."

Brittle bones are another problem of advancing years.

Bones have always fascinated archeologists because they seem to last forever. They are the last remnants after everything else is long decayed. It is the mineral portion that lasts so long. The bony skeleton may be familiar to medical students, but has spooky connotations for children of all ages. The skull and crossbones is also a traditional omen of evil and piracy, often signaling "death" or "poison" when on labels.

It's only natural to think of bone as permanent, but actually bone changes constantly throughout life. As we get older, it gradually becomes dryer, lighter and more porous. Hence the name "osteoporosis"—porous bone. However, though there is a certain normal porosity due to aging, it is sometimes hard to tell where one process ends and a pathological deficiency begins.

Osteoporosis is at once the most common, yet least understood of bone disorders. Apparently dinosaurs suffered from it, and osteoporosis has also been found in many Egyptian skeletons. In the living human, diagnosis is made by x-ray, but an x-ray will detect only gross bone changes.

Osteoporosis affects both sexes, but is at least four times more frequent in women. It affects whites earlier than Negroes, and it affects women at an earlier age than men. The disorder is associated with a thinning and weakening of bones, with a greater tendency to fracture, especially so-called compression fractures of the vertebrae. The disorder is sometimes known as "senile" or "postmenopausal" osteoporosis because of its greater frequency after the menopause. And that is why diminished estrogen production has been implicated, though exactly *how* estrogen is involved is not clear.

Actually, osteoporosis is frequently associated with other endocrine disorders—the parathyroids (hyperparathyroidism), the adrenals (Cushing's disease), the thyroid (hyperthyroidism) and the pituitary (acromegaly). To add to the confusion, osteoporosis is also associated with calcium deficiency, rheumatoid arthritis, general malnutrition, elderly patients on corticosteroid therapy and post-traumatic immobilization.

Different surveys show the incidence of osteoporosis to vary from 15 to 50 percent of the over-65 population. But most of these statistics come from old age homes and involve individuals under some sort of medical care. A figure frequently cited as an overall estimate of the incidence of this disorder postmenopausally is 25 percent of all women. More specific studies have placed the incidence somewhat higher. In any event, osteoporosis has been reevaluated as a possible pathological dysfunction rather than a normal accompaniment of the aging process.

Although some patients with definite osteoporosis have no symptoms, the most common complaint when symptoms are present is backache. This is either low or midthoracic, can be quite severe (often radiating down the legs), and is usually relieved by sitting on a straight-backed chair or by lying on a hard surface. The most common complications of decreased bone density are hip fractures and vertebral body collapse. In older patients the spine may shorten or bend due to loss of intervertebral cartilage, resulting in so-called dowager's hump.

What is the relationship between osteoporosis and estrogen deficiency? This is another controversial subject.

Arguments in favor of relating osteoporosis in the female to diminished estrogen function are of the circumstantial evidence variety: The incidence of osteoporosis is higher in postmenopausal women than in younger women; women whose ovaries are removed tend to develop the condition sooner, and more severely; treatment with estrogens usually gives relief of symptoms; a negative calcium balance can often be converted into a positive one with estrogen therapy. In one study, height loss was halted with estrogen therapy, and the number of fractures appeared to be diminished.

What have we on the other side of the ledger? Most observers agree that symptomatic relief can be provided by estrogens. But, while estrogen does produce calcium retention, there is no increased deposit of calcium, just a decrease of breakdown from the bone. In fact, whatever the mechanism of estrogen relief, there is no change at all in the x-ray picture: there is no reversal.

Moreover, the estrogen effect on the negative calcium balance seems to be nonspecific—a similar effect can be obtained with testosterone or even albumin. In addition, some studies have shown that in some patients with classic osteoporosis, administration of estrogen has practically no effect on mineral balance. Nor is there any indication of the duration of beneficial estrogen effect. Some people do not retain mineral for more than a short period of time even on high dosage of estrogen. That is, the effect often appears to wear off.

Another view of the cause of osteoporosis is that calcium loss is the culprit. Investigators point out that a low calcium intake can produce osteoporosis, more so than a protein deficiency, and that there's no proof that estrogen recalcifies bone, even if it does help the symptoms. They, therefore, feel that calcium rejection is primary, protein loss secondary. There are studies showing improvement in both mineral retention and in symptoms by feeding large amounts of calcium. Some feel that a high calcium intake is more effective than estrogen in promoting a positive calcium balance. But not all patients benefit, even though calcium needs do increase with age in both men and women.

In the case of both calcium and estrogen therapy for osteoporosis, neither method causes a reversal of the x-ray picture, though further thinning may be prevented.

Currently, experiments are being conducted with fluorides alone for osteoporosis, and there's some indication of benefit. It should be added that fluoride therapy for osteoporosis is still in the evaluation stage. Contraindications and better definition of toxic doses remain to be determined.

The various claims for the therapeutic effectiveness of different regimens for the treatment of osteoporosis leads to the concept that this bone disorder probably has *multiple* causes, resulting in increased resorption of bone. Therefore no single approach can be expected to be effective in all cases. A multifaceted approach to therapy would thus seem advisable. Good objective measures are still needed to detect this disorder in the very early stages, as well as long term follow-up studies with good controls.

Like so many other postmenopausal problems, the one posed by osteoporosis once again demonstrates that a particular finding *may* be related to estrogen deficiency. Inadequate mineral intake, poor mineral absorption and lack of physical activity are other factors which play a dominant role in many cases.

For those women who have osteoporosis, and indeed for all older women, a high protein diet with adequate vitamin D, increased calcium intake and greater physical activity are all advisable. In addition, long term estrogen therapy is justified for osteoporosis from the clinical point of view, particularly when there is pain. As Goodman and Gilman say in their classic text, such treatment is advisable, "even though one does not have the satisfaction of knowing why."

What about prevention of menopause itself?

When most doctors talk about preventing the menopause, they are talking about preventing the effects of hormonal deficiency. In this sense, menopause can be prevented. But I see no reason to start hormone therapy prior to any evidence that there is, in fact, such a deficiency. One woman at the age of 43 may show signs of definite estrogen lack. Another at 55 may as yet show none. Estrogen deficiency doesn't occur overnight. There's plenty of time to prevent the possible effects of severe prolonged deficiency by a careful medical evaluation every few months. For this and other reasons, I emphatically advise every woman to have a gynecological examination at least once a year before the age of 40 and twice a year thereafter.

Some proponents of "estrogen forever" claim that inducing cyclic bleeding for life in postmenopausal women restores their faith in their femininity. I do not agree. Although many women equate loss of menstrual function with loss of femininity and are upset by this physiological change, I have found that restoring menstrual function with hormones seldom alters that feeling. In the first place, the woman knows it is an artificial flow. Furthermore, most

147

postmenopausal women are not at all eager to resume menstruation, if given a choice.

However, the restoration of menstrual bleeding is but one method of hormonal replacement. As I've said, there are other ways of replacing estrogen which involve the production of very occasional periods, or none at all. How long to keep up such replacement therapy is an unsettled question. There are many physicians who oppose its routine use for life. It will take many years before enough scientific evidence accumulates to make a firm judgment about the advantages as well as limitations of long term hormonal therapy. Certainly *if* it is conclusively shown that any metabolic or cancerous disorders are prevented or benefited by such prolonged therapy, that will be a strong argument in favor of it. In the meantime, every physician will have to evaluate every case on its own merits. *Individualization is the key to successful therapy of the menopause and post-menopause.*

If cessation of menstrual periods happens as early as the twenties or thirties, it is necessary to find out why the ovaries are not functioning properly. This is done by checking out the thyroid, pituitary and adrenal glands. It may be that the body is producing estrogen which isn't being properly utilized. In any event, estrogen replacement is particularly important in this younger age group not only to prevent premature atrophic changes, but also because fertility may not yet be irreversible.

The "premature menopause" that may occur in the twenties or thirties is not necessarily analogous to the permanent menopause of middle age with its irreversible aging of the ovaries. When premature menopause in a younger woman is due to absence of ovulation, any medical measures which restore ovulation will also restore normal spontaneous menstrual function.

For instance, Mrs. M., a married woman of 32, and an

attractive fashion designer, had no menstrual periods for almost a year. Before that, her cycle had been irregular for many years. Since she was eager to have children, it was doubly important to discover why she was not ovulating or menstruating. An infertility workup and physical examination disclosed that she was suffering from a hormonal imbalance associated with cystic ovaries. Far from having a lack of estrogen there was, if anything, an overabundance. I prescribed an anti-estrogenic compound, which caused her to ovulate and consequently to menstruate. Some months later she conceived, and was delivered of a normal baby girl.

Another case, which sounded similar but turned out not to be, was that of an unmarried woman of 31, an executive secretary. Miss H. had had no menstrual periods for over two years. Her chief complaint was an irritation of the vagina. She hoped to marry and have children. Physical examination was negative except for a marked atrophy of the vaginal mucous membrane. An endocrinological workup revealed that the absence of her monthly periods was due to a complete ovarian failure. Although this uncommon condition is today unfortunately not amenable to restoration of ovulation, estrogen and progesterone replacement was given. This, at least, restored monthly flow. In addition, local estrogen was given for the vaginal irritation.

Not every medical problem has a completely satisfactory solution. But many do. Happily, most menstrual disturbances associated with infertility in younger women can be helped by modern methods.

Fortunately, we live in an age of enlightened, preventive medicine. We know it is more sensible to try to avoid or prevent a disorder than wait for it to develop. Many diseases that plagued our parents are now less frequent because of great progress in immunology and chemotherapy. Hopefully, our children and our grandchildren will be spared many of the disorders that afflict us today.

149

14

A Gift of Years

All would live long, but none would be old.

The attitude of primitive societies toward the elderly has varied from veneration to complete neglect. In some cultures, veneration of age extended as far as creating gods in the image of the old. The Polar Eskimo believed that the goddess Nerivik was an ancient woman who lived beneath the waters, while the Kwakiutl believed that the winds were controlled by an old woman. The Navaho "worshipped a goddess who grew old and became young again in a never-ending cycle."

In many societies when old age did carry prestige, it was enhanced by the fact that the final pronouncements of the elderly before death (whether curses or blessings) were frequently regarded as legally binding. Therefore, it was thought best to court the favor of the elderly.

Actually, the definition of "old age" has varied. A person was considered "old" whenever he or she was so regarded by contemporaries. Among the Bontoc in the Philippines, for example, a woman of thirty is already getting "old." Mongolian women are often old and wrinkled at forty. This is not to say, however, that longevity is unknown. In various tribes, there are isolated reports of ages past one hundred.

Some primitive groups gave special privileges to older women, such as making them mistresses in polygamous households. Or they were permitted to sit in on councils

151

usually reserved for men. Older women were also in demand as midwives.

In the *traditional* pattern of Chinese life, it is the moral duty of the young to support the old. In Japan, submission to parents' wishes is considered a sign of character. The Japanese recently took a conscience-stricken look at their own aged, traditionally revered, and marked September 15th the observance of a new national holiday called Keiro-No-Hi, Day of Respect to the Aged, in the hope that this gesture will stimulate improved welfare programs.

But in other cultures attitudes toward the aged was far from respectful. Under varying circumstances according to environmental and cultural conditions—severe climate, inadequate food supply, nomadic tribes on the move—the aged were neglected, cast out or even killed.

Abandonment of the elderly was common among North American Indians and was part of approved custom. Those who were too feeble to travel with the tribe were usually left at a camp to die. The old apparently did not consider this a sign of cruelty or ingratitude, but rather a sad necessity. This custom was also prevalent among the South American Amazons, the Lapp of northern Europe and the bushmen in Africa, where it was considered an act of mercy.

Sometimes suicide of the old and feeble was encouraged by custom. This was common in some of the Indian and Eskimo tribes, who believed that taking one's life was morally right "when it became heavier than death". Here again it was not a sign of cruelty but rather proof of devotion that the aged were "helped" to die.

This aversion to disability in old age was carried on to an extreme among the Aztec, who believed that the hereafter would be too gloomy for the elderly. It was therefore the custom among the Shilluk tribe to kill their own king if he showed signs of failing strength—one such sign was inability to sexually satisfy his wives. This was a little different from the custom of the Xosa, whose remedy for aging men was frequent marriages with young women.

What about the older people in our country? By 1970, there will be 20 million people 65 or over. For many, there are heavy burdens in these later years—decline in general health, loss of financial security, death of a spouse, change in environment.

Interestingly, it is commonly thought that individuals with psychological problems find them increased in old age. This has been disproved. Many seemingly well-adjusted people go to pieces with age. Yet others, whose earlier lives were marked by conflict and hardship, often find the later years singularly tranquil. Now they can be legitimately passive and dependent.

Unfortunately, our medical schools still do not emphasize the problems of chronic diseases and aging. Geriatrics is still regarded as a second-rate subject and has no specialty board of its own. It should have such a board, as a step toward the recognition of the problems of this increasing segment of the population.

One medical question that always arises when discussing the elderly is whether there is any need for estrogen at this time of life. Often there is. Women of this age are often troubled with atrophic vaginitis—itching, irritation, painful intercourse. Estrogen is in order. Occasionally the complaint at this age is vaginal prolapse, a herniation or bulge of vaginal tissue overlying the bladder or rectum, or a descent of the womb itself.

With advancing years, a woman's own estrogen stores are likely to be at their lowest. And in the older woman relatively small doses of estrogen generally suffice. In my experience, women past 65 are quite reluctant to menstruate again, and therefore the hormonal program prescribed can specifically avoid this.

Some women this age need no estrogen because they are in good physical condition and feel well. For some reason, their estrogen stores are sufficient. Others may require estrogen just locally, for vaginal tissues.

While much can be done to help the older woman feel better, nothing can stop the aging process itself. Unfortunately a great many people continue to fall prey to various fraudulent rejuvenating or health schemes. So serious has this sort of quackery become that a special Senate subcommittee on frauds, chaired by Senator Harrison A. Williams, Jr., of New Jersey, has referred to the elderly in America as a growing group of victims surrounded by sharks who take a bite roughly estimated at $1 billion a year for health quackery items and services alone! The Third National Congress on Medical Quackery, co-sponsored by the American Medical Association and the National Health Council, has discussed topics such as health food fads, obesity, cancer, mental health and psychological counseling.

Measures are indeed needed to protect aging persons from the unscrupulous peddlers of youth and revitalization that are part of our past—and present.

For example, vitamins have been widely promoted as geriatric aids, although the Council on Foods and Nutrition of the American Medical Association has stated that extra vitamins have little or no special function in geriatric therapy.

Several men recently were sentenced to prison in Iowa for mail fraud and conspiracy. They sold vitamins and food supplements on the basis of faked urinalysis reports. They claimed a hormonal imbalance was found reflecting a nutritional deficiency in the patients that could be corrected through the use of food products they sold.

The use of unusual health aids and devices probably

goes back to ancient magic. Each era seems to have both its own pitchmen and gullible buyers.

In the eighteenth century there was Friedrich Anton Mesmer who used hypnotism to "mesmerize" his subjects —but with various "scientific" touches, such as having the subject lie down on iron filings in order to "soak up magnetic fluid". He was denounced by the French Academy of Medicine, after which hypnotism fell into such disrepute that for nearly two centuries physicians practically ignored the technique.

The nineteenth century brought with it such notables as John Buchanan, who preached "animal magnetism". There was also John Campbell, inventor of "vita waves" having "healing powers". His subjects were obliged to part their hair, since the "healing waves" were supposed to enter through the scalp, and hair interfered.

Early in the twentieth century patent medicines were going great guns. There were "step right up" cure-alls everywhere. One especially clever huckster was "Doc" Ray Black. He had a foolproof formula—a very long lecture, calculated to make his standing listeners so tired that they would develop a backache right there. At this point he would elaborate his main theme, that the first sign of kidney trouble was an aching back. Sales were brisk!

Another sharp character in the early part of this century was Dr. Albert Abrams, founder of a bogus electrotherapy cult. His book, *New Concepts of Diagnosis and Treatment* published in 1922, presented concepts which were new indeed. He claimed he could make any diagnosis, even by mail, simply by putting a drop of the patient's blood (*sent to him*) on the Abrams' diagnostic machine, the "dynamizer". Wrote Abrams: "These few drops of blood carry within themselves the radioactive qualities which, when properly interpreted, convey an accurate picture of the physical condition of the patient in the same manner that the point of the needle of the phonograph carries the tones of the entire orchestra, from piccolo to bass-drum." Treatment of disease would be by vibration, using the Abrams "oscilloclast". He and his disciples reaped quite a fortune, until—

> A Chensaning, Michigan, physician . . . requested that Dr. Abrams make a diagnosis of a drop of blood on blotting paper sent by post. Doctor Abrams diagnosed the patient as having diabetes, malaria, cancer and syphilis. The blood sample he had sent in—the Michigan doctor revealed—was that of a young Plymouth Rock rooster whose virtue was unimpeachable since it had never left its cage since birth.

The American Medical Association in 1923 branded Abrams a colossal fraud. This did not stop him. However, pneumonia did.

As recently as the 1940's, a device known as the "Drown Radio Vision Instrument" was being used by its innovator, Ruth S. Drown, a chiropractor, to diagnose and treat ailments. It benefited only Mrs. Drown. She was successfully prosecuted in 1949, but she and her disciples were not out of business. Therefore, in 1963, California authorities had a housewife, a Mrs. Metcalf, send in a blood sample—of a turkey—saying it was her daughter's. Mrs. Drown's diagnosis: "The girl had chicken pox and mumps."

Less humorous are quack cancer cures. More than 500,000 Americans develop cancer every year. Books on favorable effects of unproven remedies are plentiful. They consist of false generalizations and conclusions drawn from coincidence. They prey on the victim's desire for the miraculous, and substitute emotion for fact. This is serious. Cure of cancer depends upon early diagnosis and treatment. Worthless remedies delay proper therapy.

A Gift of Years

Dr. R.N. Grant, director of professional education for the American Cancer Society, and Irene Bartlett, program associate for the Committee on New and Unproven Methods of Cancer Treatment, have recommended far-reaching extensions of public and professional education about treatment methods, as well as public meetings to expose worthless health practices. Emphasis is on the local level. Some gain has already been made. With the Kefauver-Harris amendments to the Pure Food, Drug and Cosmetics Act, the burden of proof is now on the advocates of cancer remedies.

In general, the problem of controlling unproven cancer cures is being approached on three fronts—investigation, education and legislation.

The promise of cure for arthritis is another big business that preys on the elderly. The Arthritis Foundation estimates that in 1965 arthritis victims spent about $250 million on misrepresented drugs, devices and treatments.

As long as there are gullible persons and shrewd promotors, the problem of medical quackery will exist. Among several American Medical Association pamphlets that describe this problem, one is called *The Merchants of Menace.* It warns that the old-time medicine man is still with us. Another pamphlet, *Mechanical Quackery,* shows photographs of devices used to defraud the public, just a few examples of the many used by cultists and quacks.

The 65-and-older group is increasing by some 350,000 individuals each year. It isn't that the total span of life has been prolonged, but that more and more people are attaining optimal life spans, a gift of years from medical science.

And it is precisely because so many people are living longer and reaching the category of "elderly" that good health in the *middle* years is so important.

❧

15

The Ageless Woman

Woman is the creator and fosterer of life.
ASHLEY MONTAGU

ॐ

My first professional experience with a "change of life baby" took place many years ago when I was in charge of the obstetrical service at a large Air Force base. The war was recently over, and female dependents of all military personnel were permitted to live with their husbands. My commanding officer, who was in his early sixties at the time, called me in one day and told me that his wife, age 46, was in her fourth month of pregnancy, having thought at first that she was going through the menopause. The colonel looked a little embarrassed, almost sheepish. Both he and his wife had grown children by previous marriages, and this turn of events was as bewildering as it was unexpected.

His wife viewed the news with mixed feelings. She was emotionally unprepared for the reality of the new life within her. At the same time, it did make her feel young again. Fortunately, it took the usual nine months, which gave both of them enough time to become accustomed to her new status and accept it. She had a normal delivery, and for some months afterward the colonel's home could easily be recognized by his clothesline, with its infant-wear white in the semitropical sun.

The colonel's wife was an exception. The play *Never Too Late* is on the same subject. Audiences have found it amusing, probably because of the incongruity of an un-expected "mixed blessing".

I have noticed something curious. When a woman in her forties misses a menstrual period for the first time, she urgently calls for an appointment for an examination because she's worried about pregnancy. She'll say she's heard about "change of life babies", and that she's totally unprepared for one. All this is invariably said with a smile. I think she knows, subconsciously at least, that the verdict is almost certain to be menopause. I think she asks about pregnancy because the question itself makes her feel young again. The fact that pregnancy is even a remote possibility gives a woman at least a verbal link to a childbearing age that is fast going.

So I do not emphasize the obvious. I say that examination does not substantiate her fear. At the same time, I advise that contraceptive measures be kept up one year or longer, just to be safe. I do not really think elaborate precautions are necessary as a woman approaches fifty, but the contraceptive advice is always gratefully accepted. It's reminiscent of younger years when the fear of "getting caught" was so real.

To those women who have remained childless, the menopause comes as a "final closing of the gates of hope," as Margaret Mead has said. This is as serious as it sounds, for biologically a woman's prime function is bearing children. Frustration of this role is not easy to tolerate. Studies of primitive societies have indicated that sex and reproduction permeated woman's entire personality. Plato said that even thinking was sublimation of sexuality, and in most languages the word "conceive" has the two meanings of thinking and becoming pregnant.

Actually, pregnancy after the menopause is relatively rare. There have been a number of surveys along this line, but it has been difficult to establish authentic records. One study indicated that, in general, pregnancy after 47 is "highly unlikely", another that pregnancy in women over 50 is "extremely rare". Still another review concluded that there are few authenticated records of childbirth in the 50's. In 50,000 deliveries surveyed, none of the women was over 50; two were 48, and two were 46. However, the authors point out that spontaneous abortions are more frequent in women over 40. This influences the statistics regarding full-term delivery. Another study reviewed a number of apparently authentic cases of full-term delivery in women past 50. This study noted that although the *rarity* of this event is mentioned in records of many *hospital* obstetrical services, significant numbers of such cases were found in records of vital statistics. The investigator felt that faulty recollection of age probably was responsible for this discrepancy. The overall conclusion was that the chance of pregnancy after age 50 is negligible and decreases thereafter to a vanishing point.

Nevertheless, medicolegal opinions tend to play it safe. For example, the English courts concluded that "we cannot pretend to fix the age at which pregnancy ceases to be possible, and beyond which it cannot occur." The common law in the United States concurs with the English—a woman "is conclusively presumed to be capable of children until death."

There are both anatomic and physiologic reasons for the rarity of pregnancy in women approaching 50. A young girl starts out with about half a million immature egg follicles. This number falls to about 150,000 between age 18 and 24, and to about 8,000 at age 40 to 44. If this still sounds like more than enough, keep in mind that in a whole lifetime only about 400 eggs will ever mature and be capable of being fertilized. Physiologically, even if a woman does ovulate irregularly in her late forties, the fertility of the egg is likely to be too poor for conception. Fatherhood, in contrast, can be achieved even very late in life, as we know from the experiences of various celebrities.

Let us here and now deflate the myth that the continuous use of birth control pills will cause or enable grandmothers in their sixties to have babies. When estrogens and progestins (or birth control pills, which utilize both) are given to older women for the purpose of deliberately prolonging cyclic menstrual bleeding, such artificially induced "periods" are not accompanied by ovulation and the woman remains just as infertile as she would be if no hormones were given. Hormones cannot delay aging of the ovaries. So no pregnant grandmothers are to be expected, unless they are young grandmothers to begin with.

Perhaps this is just as well. And perhaps this is one of nature's protective mechanisms. Pregnancy in the forties is associated with a slightly greater risk to woman and child, usually because of increased blood pressure associated with poor nourishment from an inadequately formed placenta. The incidence of some congenital birth defects is also somewhat higher. The woman over forty having her first baby has a greater tendency to longer labor. The cervix and vagina are not as elastic as in younger women, the uterine contractions tend to be more erratic, and the cesarean section rate is higher than for younger women.

Despite the added risk, there is no real reason to dissuade a woman in this age group from conceiving, if she wants a baby. Modern, fully equipped and fully staffed maternity units can handle just about every medical contingency.

When women stop menstruating in their forties, however, it is most often not because of pregnancy but because of menopause. Ovarian function is on the wane, and the pituitary "ovary-stimulating" hormone increases markedly in an effort to prod the less responsive ovaries. It is this high level of pituitary hormone found in the urine of postmenopausal women that has been extracted in the manufacture of a new fertility drug. The drug is used to stimulate certain types of failing ovaries of young infertile women. Many of the widely publicized cases of multiple pregnancy are due to the successful, but dramatically unpredictable, response to this hormone. In most cases, however, the result is a normal, single birth.

Thus the menopausal woman, no longer able to conceive, still possesses the gift of life. She can provide the biological stimulus to help younger, infertile women have babies.

We have come full circle back to fertility again. It is a rejuvenating thought.

❦

Bibliography

CHAPTER 1. LONGEVITY AND THE QUEST FOR
YOUTH AND BEAUTY

Acs, G. "The Biochemical Basis of Some Aspects of Heredity." *Medical Science*, 17: 47, 1966.

American Medical Association's Council on Drugs, quoted by Smith, R.L., "A Phony Fountain of Youth." *Today's Health*, 44: 27, 1966.

Clark, A.M. "Genetic Factors Associated with Aging." In: *Advances in Gerontological Research*, Strehler, B.L. (Ed.), Academic Press, New York, 1964.

Comfort, A. *The Biology of Senescence*, Rhinehart, New York, 1956.

Curtis, H.J. *Biological Mechanisms of Aging*, Charles C Thomas, Springfield, 1966.

Dublin, L.I., Lotka, A.J., and Spiegelman, M. *Length of Life: A Study of the Life Table*, Ronald Press, New York, 1949.

Editorial, "An Apple a Day?" *Medical Science*, 17: 84, 1966.

Failla, G. "The Aging Process and Carcinogenesis." *Annals of the New York Academy of Sciences*, 71: 1124, 1958.

Falek, A., *et al.* "Longevity and Intellectual Variation in a Senescent Twin Population." *Journal of Gerontology*, 15: 305, 1960.

Bibliography

Howitt, A.W. *Native Tribes of Southeast Australia*, London, 1904.

Johnson, H.D., *et al.* "Effects of 48 Degrees Farenheit and 83 Degrees Farenheit on Longevity and Pathology of Male Rats." *Journal of Gerontology*, 18: 29, 1961.

Jones, H.B. "A Special Consideration of the Aging Process, Disease and Life Expectancy." In: *Biological and Medical Physics*, Vol. 4, The Academic Press, New York, 1956.

Kral, V.A. *et al.* "Procaine (Novocaine) Treatment of Patients with Senile and Arteriosclerotic Brain Disease." *Canadian Medical Association Journal*, 87: 1109, 1962.

Lyons, L. "The Lyons Den", The New York *Post*, May 17, 1966.

Pearl, R. *Studies in Human Biology*, Williams and Wilkins. Baltimore, 1924.

Pickering, Sir G.W. "Science Moves to Counter Aging." *Medical World News*, 4: 44, 1966.

Ploss, H.H., Bartels, M., and Bartels, P. *Woman: An Historical, Gynaecological, and Anthropological Compendium*, Vols. 1 and 3, William Heinemann, Ltd., London, 1935.

Rosen, S., and Olin, P. "Hearing Loss and Coronary Heart Disease." *Archives of Otolaryngology*, 82: 236, 1965.

Scheinfeld, A. *Your Heredity and Environment*, J.B. Lippincott, Philadelphia, 1965.

Schulman, E., "Bristlecone Pine: Oldest Known Living Thing." *National Geographic Magazine*, 113: 355, 1958.

Seyle, H. *The Stress of Life*, McGraw-Hill, New York, 1956.

Shock, N., quoted by Smith, R.L. "A Phony Fountain of Youth." *Today's Health*, 44: 27, 1966.

Simmons, L.W. *The Role of the Aged in Primitive Society*, Yale University Press, 1945.

Skeat, W.W., and Blagden, C.O. *Pagan Races of the Malay Peninsula*, Vol. 2, London, 1906.

Spector, W.S. (Ed.) *Handbook of Biological Data*. W.B. Saunders Co., Philadelphia, 1961.

Sulkin, N.M., and Strevanij, P. "The Experimental Production of Senile Pigments in the Nerve Cells of Young Rats." *Journal of Gerontology*, 15: 2, 1960.

Verzar, F. "Aging of Connective Tissue." *Gerontologia*, 1: 363, 1957.

Walford, R.L. "Auto-immunity and Aging." *Journal of Gerontology*, 17: 281, 1962.

Bibliography

CHAPTER 2. CHANGE OF LIFE . . . IN A LIFE OF CHANGE

Benedick, R. "Continuities and Discontinuities in Cultural Conditioning." *Psychiatry*, 1: 161, 1938.

Currier, A.F. *The Menopause*, D. Appleton & Co., New York, 1897.

Erikson, E.H. "Growth and Crises of the Healthy Personality." *Psychological Issues*, 1: 50, 1959.

Ford, C.S., and Beach, F.A. *Patterns of Sexual Behavior*, Harper & Bros. and Paul Hoeber, New York, 1949.

Kaufman, S.A. "Current Concepts of Estrogen Replacement Therapy." Symposium, under the direction of Excerpta Medica Foundation, New York City, December 13–14, 1965.

Kaufman, S.A. "Slowing Down the Aging Process: Fact or Myth?"—Presented at the New York Academy of Sciences, October 15, 1964.

Robinson, B. "The Menopause." *Journal of the American Medical Association*, 23: 345, 1894.

Simmons, L.W. *The Role of the Aged in Primitive Society*, Yale University Press, 1945.

Von Graff, E. "Climacteric Changes." *Journal of the Iowa State Medical Society*, 22: 183, 1932.

CHAPTER 3. HORMONES, SEX GLANDS, AND MENOPAUSE

Allen, E., and Doisy, E.A. "An Ovarian Hormone. Preliminary Report on its Localization, Extraction, and Partial Purification, and Action in Test Animals." *Journal of the American Medical Association*, 81: 819, 1923.

Apostolakis, M., and Loraine, J.A. "Renal Clearance of Pituitary Gonadotropins in Postmenopausal Women." *Journal of Clinical Endocrinology*, 20: 1437, 1960.

Brown, J.B. "Urinary Excretion of Oestrogens During the Menstrual Cycle." *Lancet*, 1: 320, 1955.

Goodman, L.S., and Gilman, A. *The Pharmacological Basis of Therapeutics*, The Macmillan Co., New York, 3rd Ed., 1965.

Greenhill, J.P. "Hypothalamic (psychogenic, neurovegetative, psychosomatic) amenorrhea." *Gynecologie Pratique*, 4: 431, 1953.

Greenwood, F.C. and Bulbrook, R.D. "Effect of Hypophysectomy on Urinary Estrogen in Breast Cancer." *British Medical Journal*, 1: 666, 1957.

Bibliography

Israel, S.L. "Hypothalamic Function and Reproduction." *Obstetrics and Gynecology*, 20: 826, 1962.

Kleegman, S.J., and Kaufman, S.A. *Infertility in Women*, F.A. Davis Co., Philadelphia, 1966.

Kretzschmar, W.A., and Stoddard, F.J. "Physiological Changes in the Aging Female." *Clinical Obstetrics and Gynecology*, 7: 451, 1964.

Reynolds, S.R.M., *et al.* "Dermovascular Effects of Estrogen in Women with Menopausal Flushes." *Surgery, Gynecology, and Obstetrics*, 73: 206, 1941.

Riley, G.M. "Endocrinology of the Climacteric." *Clinical Obstetrics and Gynecology*, 7: 432, 1964.

Sturgis, S.H. "Clinical and Laboratory Diagnosis of Amenorrhea." *Gynecologie Pratique*, 4: 279, 1953.

CHAPTER 4. HOW YOU FEEL

Barrett, L. *et al.* "An Investigation of the Menopause in 1,000 Women." *Lancet*, 1: 106, 1933.

Currier, A.F. *The Menopause*, D. Appleton & Co., New York, 1897.

"Estrogens During and After the Menopause." *The Medical Letter*, 7: 54, 1965.

Gottschalk, L.A. "Psychogenic Factors in Backache." *General Practitioner*, 1: 91, 1966.

Greenblatt, R.B. "Estrogen Therapy for Postmenopausal Females." *New England Journal of Medicine*, 272: 305, 1965.

Israel, S.L. "The Menopause." *Postgraduate Medicine*, 30: 417, 1961.

Kaufman, S.A. "Relationship and Limitations of Hormonal Therapy and Maturation Index to Menopausal Symptoms." —Presented at the annual meeting of the American College of Obstetricians and Gynecologists, Washington, D.C., April 20, 1967.

Kretzschmar, W.A., and Stoddard, F.J. "Physiologic Changes in the Aging Female." *Clinical Obstetrics and Gynecology*, 7: 451, 1954.

Kupperman, H.S., *et al.* "Comparative Clinical Evaluation of Estrogenic Preparations by the Menopausal and Amenorrheal Indices." *Journal of Clinical Endocrinology*, 13: 688, 1953.

Neugarten, B.L., and Kraines, R.J. " 'Menopausal Symptoms' in Women of Various Ages." *Psychosomatic Medicine*, 27: 266, 1965.

Bibliography

Novak, E.R. "Menopause." *Journal of the American Medical Association* 156; 575, 1954.

Reynolds, S.R.M. *Physiological Bases of Gynecology and Obstetrics*, Charles C Thomas, Springfield, 1952.

Selected Questions and Answers, American Medical Association, Chicago, 1965.

CHAPTER 5. HORMONES AND CANCER

Andrews, W.C. "Estrogens and Endometrial Carcinoma." *Obstetrical and Gynecological Survey*, 16: 747, 1961.

Bishop, P.M.F. "Hormones and Cancer." *Clinical Obstetrics and Gynecology*, 3: 1109, 1960.

Blinick, G., and Kaufman, S.A. *Modern Office Gynecology*, Lea & Febiger, Philadelphia, 1957.

Emge, L.A. "Endometrial Cancer and Feminizing Tumors of Ovaries: Significance of Their Coexistence." *Obstetrics and Gynecology*, 1: 511, 1953.

Engle, E.T., and Zuckerman, S. "Effects of Prolonged Oestrin Stimulation on the Cervix Uteri." *Lancet*, 1: 435, 1937.

Gardner, W.U. "Effect of Estrogen on Incidence of Mammary and Pituitary Tumors in Hybrid Mice." *Cancer Research*, 1: 345, 1941.

Geist, S.H., and Salmon, U.J. "Are Estrogens Carcinogenic in Human Females?" *American Journal of Obstetrics and Gynecology*, 51: 29, 1941.

Gusberg, S.B. "Precursors of Corpus Carcinoma; Estrogens and Endometrial Hyperplasia." *American Journal of Obstetrics and Gynecology*, 54: 905, 1947.

Hertz, R., and Bailar, J.C. "Estrogen-Progestin Combinations for Contraception." *Journal of the American Medical Association*, 198: 1000, 1966.

Hertz, R., et al. "Observations on the Effect of Progesterone on Carcinoma of Cervix." *Journal of the National Cancer Institute*, 11: 867, 1951.

Hodgson, J.E., Dockerty, M.B., and Mussey, R.D. "Granulosa Cell Tumor of Ovary: Clinical and Pathological Report of 62 Cases." *Surgery, Gynecology and Obstetrics*, 81: 631, 1945.

Huggins, C., and Yang, N.C. "Induction and Extinction of Mammary Cancer." *Science*, 137: 257, 1962.

Israel, S.L. "Endometrial Carcinoma in Elderly Women and its Relation to Functioning Ovarian Tumors." *Geriatrics*, 14: 488, 1959.

Bibliography

Kaufman, S.A. "Current Concepts of Estrogen Replacement Therapy." Symposium, under the direction of Excerpta Medica Foundation, New York City, December 13–14, 1965.

Kaufman, S.A. "Slowing Down the Aging Process: Fact or Myth?"—Presented at the New York Academy of Sciences, October 15, 1964.

Kaufman, R.H., Abbott, W.P., and Wall, J.A. "The Endometrium Before and After Wedge Resection of the Ovaries for Stein-Leventhal Syndrome." *American Journal of Obstetrics and Gynecology,* 77: 1271, 1959.

Lacassagne, A. "Apparition de Cancers de la Mammelle Chez la Souris Male, Soumise a des Injections de Folliculine." *Compte Rendus Académie des Sciences,* 195: 630, 1932.

Larson, J.A. "Estrogens and Endometrial Carcinoma." *Obstetrics and Gynecology,* 3: 551, 1954.

Leis, H.P., Jr. "Endocrine Prophylaxis of Breast Cancer with Cyclic Estrogen and Progesterone." *International Journal of Surgery,* 45: 496, 1966.

Meissner, W.A., Sommers, S.C., and Sherman, G. "Endometrial Hyperplasia and Endometriosis Produced Experimentally by Estrogens." *Cancer,* 10: 505, 1957.

Mussey, E., and Malkasian, G.D. "Progestogen Treatment of Recurrent Carcinoma of the Endometrium." *American Journal of Obstetrics and Gynecology,* 94: 78, 1966.

Novak, E.R. "Relationship of Endometrial Hyperplasia and Adenocarcinoma of Uterine Fundus." *Journal of the American Medical Association,* 154: 217, 1954.

Report to the F.D.A. by the Advisory Committee on Obstetrics and Gynecology, Washington, D.C., 1966.

Steiner, G.J., Kistner, R.W., and Craig, J.M. "Histological Effects of Progestins on Hyperplasia and Carcinoma *in situ* of Endometrium." *Metabolism,* 14: 356, 1965.

Subcommittee on Breast and Genital Cancer. "Androgens and Estrogens in the Treatment of Disseminated Mammary Carcinoma: Retrospective Study of 944 Patients." *Journal of the American Medical Association,* 172: 1271, 1960.

Urban, J.A. "Current Trends in Breast Cancer Treatment." *New York State Journal of Medicine,* 61: 3120, 1961.

Wellenbach, B.L., and Rakoff, A.W. "Hyperplasia of Endometrium." *Journal of the Albert Einstein Medical Center,* 2: 3, 1953.

Wilson, R.A., "The Roles of Estrogen and Progesterone in

Breast and Genital Cancer." *Journal of the American Medical Association*, 182: 327, 1962.

CHAPTER 6. ESTROGEN REPLACEMENT THERAPY

Barnes, A.C. "The Menopause." *Clinical Obstetrics and Gynecology*, 1: 203, 1958.

Beecham, C. "Current Concepts of Estrogen Replacement Therapy." Symposium under the direction of Excerpta Medica Foundation, New York City, December 13–14, 1965.

Chang, Y.C., and Craig, J.M. "Vaginal Smear Assessment of Estrogen Activity in Endometrial Carcinoma." *Obstetrics and Gynecology*, 21: 170, 1963.

Greenblatt, R.B. "Estrogen Therapy for Postmenopausal Females" *New England Journal of Medicine*, 272: 305, 1965.

Hammond, D.O. "Endocrine Vaginal Cytology." *General Practitioner*, 30: 123, 1964.

Liu, W. *An Introduction to Gynecological Exfoliative Cytology*, Charles C Thomas, Springfield, 1959.

Kaufman, S.A. "Current Concepts of Estrogen Replacement Therapy." Symposium, under the direction of Excerpta Medica Foundation, New York City, December 13–14, 1965.

Kaufman, S.A. "Estrogen Replacement Therapy and its Metabolic Effects." Symposium, under the direction of the Council for Interdisciplinary Communication in Medicine, New York City, April 6, 1967.

Kaufman, S.A. "Relationship and Limitations of Hormonal Therapy and Maturation Index to Menopausal Symptoms." —Presented at the annual meeting of the American College of Obstetricians and Gynecologists, Washington, D.C., April 20, 1967.

Kaufman, S.A. "Slowing Down the Aging Process: Fact or Myth?"—Presented at the New York Academy of Sciences, October 15, 1964.

Navab, A., Koss, L.G., and LaDue, J.S. "Estrogen-like Activity on the Squamous Epithelium of the Female Genital Tract." *Journal of the American Medical Association*, 194: 30, 1965.

Novak, E.R., Jones, G.S., and Jones, H.W., Jr. *Textbook of Gynecology* (7th Ed.), Williams and Wilkins Co., Baltimore, 1965.

Overstreet, E.W. "Endocrine Management of the Geriatric

Woman." *American Journal of Obstetrics and Gynecology*, 95: 354, 1966.

Papanicolaou, G.N. "The Sexual Cycle in the Human Female as Revealed by Vaginal Smears." *American Journal of Anatomy*, 52: 519, 1933.

Pearl, M.J., and Plotz, E.J. "Management of the Climacteric." *Clinical Obstetrics and Gynecology*, 7: 476, 1964.

Pouchet, F.A. *Théorie Positive de l'Ovulation Spontanée et de la Fécondation*, Paris, 1847.

Randall, C.L. "Ovarian Function in Women After Menopause." *American Journal of Obstetrics and Gynecology*, 73: 1000, 1957.

Rhoades, F.P. "The Menopause, A Deficiency Disease." *Michigan Medicine*, 64: 410, 1965.

Stockard, C.R., and Papanicolaou, G.N. "The Existence of a Typical Oestrous Cycle in the Guinea-Pig—With a Study of its Histological and Physiological Changes." *American Journal of Anatomy*, 22: 225, 1917.

Sturgis, S.H. "The Challenge of Comprehensive Gynecology." *American Journal of Obstetrics and Gynecology*, 73: 180, 1957.

Wachtel, E. *Exfoliative Cytology in Gynaecological Practice*, Butterworth & Co., Ltd., London, 1964.

Wied, G.L. "Terminology of Cytologic Reporting in Endocrinological Conditions." *Acta Cytologica*, 8: 383, 1964.

Wilson, R.A., Brevetti, R.E., and Wilson, T.A. "Specific Procedures for the Elimination of the Menopause." *Western Journal of Surgery, Obstetrics and Gynecology*, 71: 110, 1963.

CHAPTER 7. THE ESTROGEN DEBATE

Danforth, D.W. "The Climacteric." *Medical Clinics of North America*, 45: 47, 1961.

Davis, M.E. "Modern Management of Menopausal Patient." *Current Medical Digest*, 33: 39, 1966.

Eichner, E. "Symptomatic Response in the Climacteric to Autonomic Stabilization." *Obstetrics and Gynecology Digest*, 7: 41, 1965.

"Estrogens During and After the Menopause." *The Medical Letter*, 7: 54, 1965.

Greenblatt, R.B., "Current Concepts of Estrogen Replacement Therapy." Symposium, under the direction of Excerpta Medica Foundation, New York City, December 13–14, 1965.

Bibliography

Jeffcoate, T.N.A. "Drugs for Menopausal Symptoms." *British Medical Journal*, 1: 340, 1960.

Kaufman, S.A. "Current Concepts of Estrogen Replacement Therapy." Symposium, under the direction of Excerpta Med-Medica Foundation, New York City, December 13–14, 1965.

Kaufman, S.A. "Family Planning in Large Indigent Population." Excerpta Medica International Congress Series No. 109, June, 1966.

Kaufman, S.A. "Limited Relationship of Maturation Index to Estrogen Therapy of Menopausal Symptoms: An Analysis of 200 Patients." *Obstetrics and Gynecology* (in preparation).

Kaufman, S.A. "Slowing Down the Aging Process: Fact or Myth?"—Presented at the New York Academy of Sciences, October 15, 1964.

Report to the F.D.A. by the Advisory Committee on Obstetrics and Gynecology, Washington, D.C., 1966.

Rhoades, F.P. "Aggressive Management of Disorders of the Aging Female." *Journal of the American Geriatrics Society*, 12: 9, 1964.

Rock, J. "Let's Be Honest About the Pill!" *Journal of the American Medical Association*, 192: 401, 1965.

Tilt, E.J. "On Uterine Pathology at the Change of Life and After the Menopause." *British Medical Journal*, 2: 435, 1870.

Von Graff, E. "Climacteric Changes" *Journal of the Iowa State Medical Society*, 22: 183, 1932.

Wilson, R.A., and Wilson, T.A. "The Fate of the Non-Treated Postmenopausal Woman: A Plea for the Maintenance of Adequate Estrogen from Puberty to the Grave." *Journal of the American Geriatrics Society*, 11: 347, 1965.

CHAPTER 8. BEAUTY AND MIDDLE AGE

Baker, T.J., and Gordon, H.L. "Chemical Face Peeling: An Adjunct to Surgical Facelifting." *Southern Medical Journal*, 56: 412, 1963.

Behrman, H.T. "Hormone Creams and Facial Skin." *Journal of the American Medical Association*, 155: 119, 1954.

Bigsby, F., and Cayetto, M. "Exercise in Obesity—Practical Considerations." *Illinois Medical Journal* 127: 680, 1965.

Braley, S. "Use of Silicones in Plastic Surgery." *Archives of Otolaryngology*, 78: 669, 1963.

Conway, H. "Weight of the Breasts as a Handicap to Respiration." *American Journal of Surgery*, 103: 674, 1962.

Bibliography

Conway, H., and Smith, J. "Breast Plastic Surgery." *Plastic and Reconstructive Surgery*, 21: 8, 1958.

Ehret, A. *Mucusless Diet Healing System*, Ehret Literature Publishing Co., Los Angeles, 1924.

Erich, J.B. "Augmentation Mammaplasty." *Mayo Clinic Proceedings*, 40: 397, 1965.

Editorial, "Abreast of the Times." *Journal of the American Medical Association*, 195: 863, 1966.

Editorial, "Skin and Sun Tanning." *New York State Journal of Medicine*, 66: 2008, 1966.

"Estrogens During and After the Menopause." *The Medical Letter*, 7: 54, 1965.

"Facts About Drugs and Devices for Weight Reduction." Miscellany. *Journal of the American Medical Association*, 171: 1731, 1960.

Goldfarb, A.F., "Hirsutism: Causes and Treatment." *Medical Science*, 17: 42, 1966.

Goldzieher, M.A. "Effects of Estrogens on Senile Skin." *Journal of Gerontology* 1: 196, 1946.

Goldzieher, M.A. "Female Sex Hormones in Practice." Clinical Seminar, Atlantic City, June 15, 1963.

Heath, R.G. *The Role of Pleasure in Behavior*, Hoeber Medical Division, Harper & Row, New York, 1964.

Kligman, A.M. "Pathologic Dynamics of Human Hair Loss." *American Medical Association Archives of Dermatology*, 83: 175, 1961.

Lubowe, I.I. "Modern Management of Hair and Scalp Disorders." *New York State Journal of Medicine*, 66: 1318, 1966.

Montagu, A. "Obesity and Evolution in Man," *Journal of the American Medical Association*, 195: 105, 1965.

Montagu, A. "The Buttocks and Natural Selection." *Journal of the American Medical Association*, 198: 169, 1966.

Obesity and Health, Mayer, J. (Ed.), U.S. Government Printing Office, Washington, D.C.

Ploss, H.H., Bartels, M., and Bartels, P. *Woman: An Historical, Gynaecological and Anthropological Compendium*, William Heinemann, Ltd., London, 1935.

Smith, R.L. "The Face Burners." *Today's Health*, 44: 20, 1966.

Strang, J.M. "Obesity." In: *Diseases of Metabolism*, Duncan, G.G. (Ed.) 4th Edition, W.B. Saunders Co., Philadelphia, 1959.

Winer, L.H., *et al.* "Tissue Reactions to Injected Silicone Liquids." *Archives of Dermatology*, 90: 588, 1964.

Bibliography

CHAPTER 9. SICK AT HEART

Alden, C.B., *et al.* "Headache." Panel discussion, *New York State Journal of Medicine,* 66: 467, 1966.

Alvarez, W.C. "The Many Causes of Migraine in Middle-Aged and Elderly Women." *Geriatrics,* 14: 433, 1959.

Blinder, M.G. "Differential Diagnosis and Treatment of Depressive Disorders." *Journal of the American Medical Association,* 195: 98, 1966.

Blinick, G., and Kaufman, S.A. *Modern Office Gynecology,* Lea & Febiger, Philadelphia, 1957.

Brocklesby, R. *Reflections on Ancient and Modern Music,* 1749.

Burton, R. *The Anatomy of Melancholy,* 1621.

Committee on Alcoholism and Council on Mental Health, "Dependence on Amphetamines and Other Stimulant Drugs." *Journal of the American Medical Association,* 197: 1023, 1966.

Current Research on Sleep and Dreams, U.S. Department of Health, Education and Welfare, Washington, D.C.

Diamond, S., "Masks of Depression." *Clinical Medicine,* 72: 1629, 1965.

Gusberg, S.B. Editorial, "Dynamic Chastity and the Copulation Explosion." *Obstetrics and Gynecology,* 28: 139, 1966.

Kroger, W.S., and Freed, S.C. *Psychosomatic Gynecology,* The Free Press, Glencoe, 1956.

Luce, G.G., and Segal, J. *Sleep,* Coward-McCann, New York, 1966.

Mannes, Marya, "The Roots of Anxiety in the Modern Woman." Symposium on anxiety, *Journal of Neuropsychiatry,* 5: 412, 1964.

McCandless, F.D. "Emotional Problems of the Climacteric." *Clinical Obstetrics and Gynecology,* 7: 489, 1964.

Shakespeare, W. *The Winter's Tale,* Act 3, Scene 3.

Socrates, quoted by Chafetz, M.E. In: *Liquor—Servant of Man,* Little, Brown & Co., Boston, 1965.

Stevens, H. "Humor Plus Humility Equals Humaneness." *Journal of the American Medical Association,* 190: 1114, 1964.

Sturgis, S.H. "Psychiatric Aspects of Gynecologic Care." *Journal of the Michigan State Medical Society,* 56: 1275, 1957.

Weiss, E., and English, O.S. *Psychosomatic Medicine* (3rd Ed.), W.B. Saunders Co., Philadelphia, 1957.

Bibliography

Wolff, H.G. *Headache and Other Head Pain* (2nd Ed.), Oxford University Press, New York, 1963.

CHAPTER 10. TO BE A WOMAN

Greenhill, J.P., and Freed, S.C. "The Mechanism and Treatment of Premenstrual Distress with Ammonium Chloride." *Endocrinology*, 26: 529, 1940.

Israel, S.L., and Weber, L.L. "Postmenopausal Uterine Bleeding." *Obstetrics and Gynecology*, 7: 286, 1956.

Kaufman, S.A., and Blinick, G. "Abnormal Vaginal Bleeding." *American Journal of Surgery*, 88: 546, 1954.

Menzer-Benaron, D., Morris, T.A., Sabbath, J., Ludwig, A.O., and Sturgis, S.H. In: *The Gynecologic Patient*, Sturgis, S.H. (Ed.), Grune & Stratton, 1962.

Morton, J.H. "Premenstrual Tension." *American Journal of Obstetrics and Gynecology*, 60: 343, 1950.

Novak, E.R. "Postmenopausal Bleeding." *Clinical Obstetrics and Gynecology*, 7: 464, 1964.

Oleck, H.L. "Legal Aspect of Premenstrual Tension." *International Records of Medicine*, 166: 492, 1953.

Paulson, M.J. "Psychological Concomitants of Premenstrual Tension." *American Journal of Obstetrics and Gynecology*, 81: 733, 1961.

CHAPTER 11. PLEASURE WITHOUT PAIN

Amelar, R.D. *Infertility in Men*, F.A. Davis Co., Philadelphia, 1966.

Bassan, J., Frame, B., and Frost, H. "Osteoporosis: A Review of Pathogenesis and Treatment." *Annals of Internal Medicine*, 58: 539, 1963.

Blinick, G., and Kaufman, S.A. *Modern Office Gynecology*, Lea & Febiger, Philadelphia, 1957.

Blinick, G., and Kaufman, S.A. "The Office Management of Leukorrhea." *American Journal of Surgery*, 85: 27, 1953.

Carrighar, S. *Wild Heritage*, Houghton Mifflin Co., Boston, 1965.

Dickinson, R.L., and Beam, L.A. *A Thousand Marriages*, Williams and Wilkins, Baltimore, 1931.

Falk, H.C., and Kaufman, S.A. "What Constitutes a Normal Semen?" *Fertility and Sterility*, 1: 489, 1950.

Bibliography

Ford, C.S., and Beach, F.A. *Patterns of Sexual Behavior*, Harper & Bros., N.Y., 1951.

Goodman, L.S., and Gilman, A. *The Pharmacological Basis of Therapeutics*, The Macmillan Co., New York, 3rd Ed., 1965.

Hampson, J.G., and Money, J. "Idiopathic Sexual Precocity in the Female." *Psychosomatic Medicine*, 17: 16, 1955.

Israel, S.L. "The Art of Caring for Women." *Journal of the American Medical Association*, 191: 393, 1965.

Kaufman, S.A. "Slowing Down the Aging Process: Fact or Myth?"—Presented at the New York Academy of Sciences, October 15, 1964.

Kaufman, S.A. "What is a Normal Semen?" *Human Fertility*, 11: 3, 1946.

Kavinoky, N., "Counseling the Marital and Sexual Problems of Older Patients." In: *Counseling in Marital and Sexual Problems: A Physician's Handbook*, Klemer, R.H. (Ed.), Williams and Wilkins, Baltimore, 1965.

Kinsey, A.C., Pomeroy, W.B., and Martin, C.E. *Sexual Behavior in the Human Male*, W.B. Saunders Co., Philadelphia, 1948.

Kinsey, A.C., Pomeroy, W.B., Martin, C.E., and Gebhard, P.H. *Sexual Behavior in the Human Female*, W.B. Saunders Co., Philadelphia, 1953.

Kleegman, S.J., and Kaufman, S.A. *Infertility in Women*, F.A. Davis Co., Philadelphia, 1966.

Kubie, L.S. In: Eisenstein, V.W. *Neurotic Interaction in Marriage*, Basic Books, New York, 1956.

Lorenz, K. *On Aggression*, Harcourt, Brace and World, Inc., New York, 1966.

MacLeod, J. "A Possible Factor in the Etiology of Human Infertility: Preliminary Report." *Fertility and Sterility*, 13: 29, 1962.

Masters, W.H., and Johnson, V.E. *Human Sexual Response*, Little, Brown & Co., Boston, 1966.

McCandless, F.D. "Emotional Problems of the Climacteric" *Clinical Obstetrics and Gynecology*, 7: 489, 1964.

Meema, H.E., Bunker, M.L., and Meema, S. "Loss of Compact Bone Due to Menopause." *Obstetrics and Gynecology*, 26: 333, 1965.

Nash, E.B., Jessner, L., and Abse, D.W. *Marriage Counseling in Medical Practice*, University of North Carolina Press, Chapel Hill, 1964.

Newman, G., and Nichols, C.R. "Sexual Activities and Atti-

Bibliography

tudes of Older Persons." *Journal of the American Medical Association*, 173: 33, 1960.

Nordin, B.E.C., *et al.* "Incidence of Osteoporosis in Normal Women: Relation to Age and Menopause." *Quarterly Journal of Medicine*, 35: 24, 1966.

Reifenstein, E.C., Jr., "The Relationship of Steroid Hormones to the Development and Management of Osteoporosis in Aging People." *Clinical Orthopedics*, 10: 206, 1957.

Robinson, B. "The Menopause" *Journal of the American Medical Association*, 23: 345, 1894.

Segal, S.J., Davidson, O.W., and Kada, K. "Role of RNA in Regulatory Action of Estrogen." *Proceedings of the National Academy of Sciences*, 54: 782, 1965.

Selle, W.A., and Jurist, J.M. "The Onset of Postmenopausal Osteoporosis as Studied by a New Technique." *Journal of the American Geriatrics Society*, 14: 930, 1966.

Seymour, F.I., Duffy, C., and Koerner, A. "A Case of Authenticated Fertility in a Man of 94." *Journal of the American Medical Association*, 105: 1423, 1935.

Sturgis, S.H. "Psychiatric Aspects of Gynecologic Care." *Journal of the Michigan State Medical Society*, 56: 1275, 1957.

Wallach, S., and Henneman, P.H. "Prolonged Estrogen Therapy in Postmenopausal Women." *Journal of the American Medical Association*, 171: 1637, 1959.

CHAPTER 12. WHEN SURGERY IS NEEDED

DeCosta, E.J. "After Office Hours: 'Dance Me Loose'" *Obstetrics and Gynecology*, 6: 120, 1955.

Douglas, G.W., and Studdiford, W.E., Jr., "Major Gynecological Surgery in the Aged Patient." *American Journal of Obstetrics and Gynecology*, 68: 456, 1954.

Falk, H.C., and Kaufman, S.A. "Partial Colpocleisis: The Le Fort Procedure; Analysis of One Hundred Cases." *Obstetrics and Gynecology*, 5: 617, 1955.

Israel, S.L. "Persistent Challenge of Hysterectomy." *Southern Medical Journal*, 58: 608, 1965.

Jones, H.W., Jr., "Stress Incontinence." *Obstetrical and Gynecological Survey*, 20: 351, 1965.

Journal of the American Medical Association, 196: 17, 1966, quoting the May 2, 1891 issue.

Kroger, W.S., and Freed, S.C. *Psychosomatic Gynecology*, The Free Press, Glencoe, 1956.

178

Bibliography

Mattingly, R.F. "Surgery in the Aging Female." *Clinical Obstetrics and Gynecology,* 7: 573, 1964.

Randall, C.L. "Ovarian Function in Women After Menopause." *American Journal of Obstetrics and Gynecology,* 73: 1000, 1957.

Randall, C.L., Birtch, P.K., and Harkins, J.L. "Ovarian Function After Menopause" *American Journal of Obstetrics and Gynecology,* 74: 719, 1957.

Sturgis, S.H., and Robey, H.S. "The Pre-operative Social Service Interview: Psychological Implications of Hysterectomy." *Connecticut Medical Journal,* 23, 786, 1959.

Tancer, M.L., and Matseone, S.L. "Gynecological Surgery in Patients over 65." *Geriatrics,* 21: 189, 1966.

TeLinde, R.W. *Operative Gynecology,* (3rd Ed.), Lippincott, Philadelphia, 1962.

CHAPTER 13. PREVENTION IS BEST

Albright, F., Smith, P.H., and Richardson, A.M. "Postmenopausal Osteoporosis—its Clinical Features." *Journal of the American Medical Association,* 116: 2465, 1941.

Alexander, J.K. "Chronic Heart Disease Due to Obesity." *Journal of Chronic Diseases,* 18: 895, 1965.

Ayre, J.E. "Vaginal Smear: 'Precancer' Cell Studies Using Modified Technique." *American Journal of Obstetrics and Gynecology,* 58: 1205, 1949.

Berkson, D.M., Stamler, J., and Cohen, D.B. "Ovarian Function and Coronary Atherosclerosis." *Clinical Obstetrics and Gynecology,* 7: 504, 1964.

Blinick, G., and Kaufman, S.A. *Modern Office Gynecology,* Lea & Febiger, Philadelphia, 1957.

"Calcium, Steroids and Osteoporosis." *The Medical Letter,* 5: 73, 1963.

Casdorph, H.R. "Fats in the Diet." *Geriatrics,* 20: 168, 1965.

Cohen, P. and Gardener, F.H. "Induction of Skeletal Fluorosis in Two Common Demineralizing Disorders." *Journal of the American Medical Association,* 195: 962, 1966.

Davis, M.E., Strandford, N.M., and Lanzl, L.H. "Estrogens and the Aging Process—The Detection, Prevention and Retardation of Osteoporosis." *Journal of the American Medical Association,* 196: 129, 1966.

Dock, W. "How Some Hearts Age." *Journal of the American Medical Association,* 195, 422, 1966.

Bibliography

Douglas, G.W., and Studdiford, W.E. Jr. "Diagnosis of Early Carcinoma of Cervix." *Surgery, Gynecology and Obstetrics,* 91: 728, 1950.

Dymling, J.F., Isaksson, B., and Sjogren, B. "Anabolic Steroids in the Treatment of Osteopenia" In: *Protein Metabolism,* Gross, F. (Ed.), Heidelberg, Springer Verlag, 1962.

Furman, R.H. "Are Gonadal Hormones (Estrogens and Androgens) of Significance in the Development of Ischemic Heart Disease?"—Presented at the New York Academy of Sciences Symposium, Conference on Atherosclerosis; Recent Developments, New York, November 22, 1966.

Gershon-Cohen, J., Haberman, J.D., Berger, S.M., and Barnes, R.B. "Newer Techniques in the Detection and Diagnosis of Breast Cancer: Mammography and Thermography." In: *Fifth National Cancer Proceedings,* J.B. Lippincott Co., Philadelphia, 1964.

Goodman, L.S., and Gilman, A. *The Pharmacological Basis of Therapeutics,* The Macmillan Co., New York, 3rd Ed., 1965.

Greene, T.H., Jr., *Gynecology: Essentials of Clinical Practice,* Little, Brown & Co., Boston, 1965.

Hecht, E.L., and Oppenheim, A. "Cytology of Endometrial Cancer." *Surgery, Gynecology and Obstetrics,* 122: 1025, 1966.

Higano, N., Robinson, R.W., and Cohen, W.D. "Increased Incidence of Cardiovascular Disease in Castrated Women. Two-Year Follow-up Studies." *New England Journal of Medicine,* 268: 1123, 1963.

Howard, A.N. *Medical Tribune,* 7: 1, 1966.

Kannel, W.B., *et al.* "Factors of Risk in the Development of Coronary Heart Disease—Six-Year Follow-Up Experience: The Framingham Study." *Annals of Internal Medicine,* 55: 33, 1961.

Kaufman, S.A. "Carcinoma of the Endometrium." *New York State Journal of Medicine,* 52: 1043, 1952.

Kaufman, S.A. "Relationship and Limitations of Hormonal Therapy and Maturation Index to Menopausal Symptoms." Presented at the annual meeting, American College of Obstetricians and Gynecologists, Washington, D.C., April 20, 1967.

Kleegman, S.J., and Kaufman, S.A. *Infertility in Women,* F.A. Davis Co., Philadelphia, 1966.

Koss, L.G. "The Present Status of Cytology in Uterine Cancer." *Ca* (American Cancer Society), 16: 198, 1966.

Bibliography

Kottke, F.J. "The Effects of Limitation of Activity Upon the Human Body." *Journal of the American Medical Association,* 196: 117, 1966.

Lutwak, L., and Whedon, G.D. "Osteoporosis" In: *Disease a Month,* Year Book Publishers, Inc., Chicago, April, 1963.

Marmorston, J., *et al.* "Effect of Premarin on Survival in Men with Myocardial Infarction." *Proceedings of the Society for Experimental Biology and Medicine,* 80: 868, 1960.

Novak, E.R., and Williams, T.J. "Autopsy Comparison of Cardiovascular Changes in Castrated and Normal Women." *American Journal of Obstetrics and Gynecology,* 80: 868, 1960.

Oliver, M.F., and Boyd, G.S. "Effects of Bilateral Ovariectomy on Coronary Artery Disease and Serum Lipid Levels." *Lancet,* 1: 690, 1959.

Oliver, M.F., and Boyd, G.S. "The Influence of Reduction of Serum Lipids on Prognosis of Coronary Heart Disease—A Five Year Study Using Estrogen." *Lancet,* 2: 499, 1961.

Papanicolaou, G.N., and Traut, H.F. *Diagnosis of Uterine Cancer by the Vaginal Smear,* The Commonwealth Fund, New York, 1943.

Pearl, M.J., and Plotz, E.J. "Management of the Climacteric." *Clinical Obstetrics and Gynecology,* 7: 476, 1964.

Perloff, W.H., and Schneeberg, N.G. "The Premature Climacterium." *American Practitioner and Digest of Treatment,* 8: 1955, 1957.

Ritterband, A.B. *et al.* "Gonadal Function and the Development of Coronary Heart Disease." *Circulation,* 27: 237, 1963.

Shapiro, S., Strax, P., and Venet, L. "Evaluation of Periodic Breast Cancer Screening with Mammography." *Journal of The American Medical Association,* 195: 731, 1966.

Stamler, J., *et al.* "Effectiveness of Estrogens for Therapy of Myocardial Infarction in Middle-Aged Men." *Journal of the American Medical Association,* 183: 632, 1963.

CHAPTER 14. A GIFT OF YEARS

Abrams, A. *New Concepts in Diagnosis and Treatment,* Physico-Clinical Co., San Francisco, 1922.

Frazer, J.G. *The Golden Bough: A Study in Magic and Religion,* New York, 1927.

Grant, R.N., and Bartlett, I. "Unproven Cancer Remedies—A Primer." *Ca* (American Cancer Society), 16: 42, 1966.

Bibliography

Rogatz, P. "Medical and Social Needs of the Aging." *New York State Journal of Medicine*, 66: 531, 1966.

Schifferes, J.J. *The Older People In Your Life*, The Washington Square Press, New York, 1962.

Simmons, L.W. *The Role of the Aged in Primitive Society*, Yale University Press, 1945.

CHAPTER 15. THE AGELESS WOMAN

Deutch, H. *The Psychology of Women*, Vol. 2, Grune & Stratton, New York, 1945.

Leach, W.B. "Perpetuity in a Nutshell." *Harvard Law Review*, 51: 683, 1938.

Mead, M. *Male and Female: A Study of the Sexes in a Changing World*, William Morrow & Co., New York, 1949.

Gemzell, C. "Human Gonadotropins in Sterility." *Fertility and Sterility*, 17: 149, 1966.

Goldberg, B.Z., *The Sacred Fire: The Story of Sex in Religion*, University Books, Inc., New York, 1958.

Kleegman, S.J., and Kaufman, S.A. *Infertility in Women*, F.A. Davis Co., Philadelphia, 1966.

Newell, J.W., and Rock, J. "Upper Age Limit of Parturition: A Review of the Literature." *American Journal of Obstetrics and Gynecology*, 63: 875, 1952.

Posner, L.B., Chidlac, J.E., and Posner, A.C. "Pregnancy at Age 40 and Over." *Obstetrics and Gynecology*, 17: 194, 1961.

Taylor, A.S. *Medical Jurisprudence*, Fifth American Edition, from Seventh London Edition, Blanchard & Lea, Philadelphia, 1861.

INDEX

Abdominal discomfort, 102
Abortion, 71
Abrams, Dr. Albert, 155–156
Acne, 71, 78
Acromegaly, 144
ACTH (adrenocorticotropic pituitary hormone), 81
Adrenal glands, 10, 23, 25, 26, 28, 52, 76, 144, 148
Adrenaline, 25, 81
Aging mechanism, biological theories of, 4–7
Ainu, 1
Air pollution, 4
Albumin, 145
Allen, Dr. Edgar, 26
Allergies, 6, 98, 102
Amazon Indians, 152
American Cancer Society, 43, 135, 157
American Medical Association, 9, 82, 154, 155, 157
Amphetamines, 98
Anatomy of Melancholy, The, 89
Androgen, 25, 52, 73, 78, 122
Anemia, 98
Anthropology, 20
Aphrodisiacs, 121
Apollo, 89
Arteries, *see* Atherosclerosis
Arthritis, 39, 157
  rheumatoid, 41, 144

Arthritis Foundation, 157
Ashanti tribe, 17
Aslan, Dr. Ana, 9
Aspirin, 37, 40, 99
Atherosclerosis, 138, 139, 141, 142
Atrophic vaginitis, 11, 31, 38, 58, 87, 111–115, 118, 129, 130, 153
Atrophy, mucosal, 59
Australian aborigines, 1
Aztec Indians, 152

Bach, Johann Sebastian, 89
Backache, 21, 38, 88, 102, 110, 144–145
Baker, Russell, 77
Baldness, 123–124
Bartlett, Irene, 157
Berbers, 1
Bible, 1, 89
Biopsy, 107, 133, 134
Birth control pills, 26, 45, 49, 52, 70–71, 78, 80, 85, 108, 162
Black, "Doc" Ray, 155
Bladder, 30, 59, 118, 129, 130, 153
Bleeding:
  abnormal, 53, 61–62, 69, 71, 72, 106–110, 112, 126, 128, 134
  cyclic menstrual, 29, 104, 162
Bloating, 101, 140
Blood pressure:

Index

Blood pressure (*cont.*)
high, 30, 34, 64, 95, 138, 141
low, 4, 95
Blood vessels, 6, 74
Bones, brittle, *see* Osteoporosis
Bontoc tribe, 151
Boredom, 97, 100
Boyish Form Brassiere Company, 84
Brain, 24, 31
See also Hypothalamus
Breasts, 26, 29–30, 57, 83–88, 90, 91, 125
cancer of, 43–45, 46–48, 49, 71
fibrocystic disease of, 47, 63
self-examination of, 135–136
soreness and swelling of, 69, 102, 110, 140
Bristlecone pine trees, 2
Brown-Séquard, Charles E., 8
Buchanan, John, 155
Burma, 12
Bursitis, 54
Bushmen, 152

Caesarean section, 162
Caffeine, 99
Campbell, John, 155
Calcium deficiency, 144, 146
Calcium theory of aging, 6
Calcium therapy, 39
Calories, 81
Cancer, 5, 17, 61, 106–107, 108, 133, 154, 156
breast, 26, 43–45, 46–48, 49, 71, 135–137
cervical, 48, 133, 134
ovarian, 48, 134
quack cures for, 156
uterine, 44, 45–46, 54, 127
Carbohydrates, 142
Casals, Pablo, 2
Cervical canal, 30
Cervical secretion, 61, 70, 71
Cervix, 48, 62, 107, 108, 125, 133–134, 162
Chagall, Marc, 2
Chemosurgery, 78, 79
Chevalier, Maurice, 11
Childbearing, 28–29, 92, 94, 97, 104, 149, 159–163
Chinese, 4, 12, 152
Chippewa Indians, 1

Cholesterol, 4, 141–142
Chorionic gonadotropin, 27
Chukchi tribe, 84
Churchill, Winston, 2
Climacteric, 15–16, 65
See also Menopause
Clover, Australian, 26
Collagen theory of aging, 5
Committee on New and Unproven Methods of Cancer Treatment, 157
Constipation, 82
Contraceptives:
oral, *see* Birth control pills
other, 72, 105, 116, 160
Contraindications to therapy, 40, 70, 72
Coronary disease, *see* Heart disease
Corpus luteum, 27
Corticosteroid therapy, 144
Cortisone, 25, 41
Creek Indians, 17
Crete, ancient, 84
Cretinism, 25
Crow Indians, 2
Crying spells, 91
Curettage, 62, 69, 107, 109, 110, 134
Cushing's disease, 144
Cystic mastitis, 69
Cystitis, *see* Bacterial infection
Cystocele, 129
Cysts:
breast, 69, 137
ovarian, 128, 149
Cytology, 52, 53, 133, 137

"D and C," *see* Curettage
Deafness, 9
Death rates, 5
Department of Foods and Nutrition of A.M.A., 82
Depression, 54, 60, 61, 63, 89–95
Dermabrasion, 78
Diabetes, 25, 53, 54, 131, 138, 141, 142, 156
Dieri tribe, 2
Diet, 98, 147
and heart disease, 142
in middle age, 79–83, 88
Digitalis, 53

186

Index

Hearing, 4
Heart, 137–143
Heart disease, 3, 4, 5, 9, 53, 54, 70,
    71, 131, 137–143
Heat therapy, 40
Hebrews, ancient, 1
Heredity, 3, 7, 12
Herniation, 129–132, 153
Hope, Bob, 7
Hormonal changes in women, 16–
    17, 25–31
Hormonal theory of aging, 6–7
Hormone therapy, 51–64
Hormones, 6, 18, 21, 23–31, 43, 48,
    51–64, 65–72
    See also Cortisone, Estrogen,
    Insulin, Progesterone, Testos-
    terone, and Thyroid
Hottentots, 2
"Housemaid's knee," 40
Hydrocortisone, 40
Hyperparathyroidism, 144
Hyperplasia, 45–46
Hypertension, 9, 131
Hypothalamus, 10, 24, 28, 29, 35,
    81
Hyperthyroidism, 144
Hysterectomy, 54, 63, 121, 125–127
Hysterogram, 107

Impotence, 9, 82, 130, 140
Index, estrogen, 51–56
India, 4
Insanity, 17
Insomnia, 11, 21, 34, 38, 57, 59, 90,
    91, 92, 95–96, 102, 118
Insulin, 25, 81
Iron, 98
Irritability, 34, 54, 102

Japanese, 152
Johnson, Virginia E., 119
*Journal of the American Medical
    Association*, 18, 40, 132

Keiro-No-Hi (Day of Respect to the
    Aged), 152
Kidneys, 10, 30
    disorders of, 5, 70, 142

Kinsey, Dr. Alfred C., 123
Koss, Dr. Leopold G., 133
Kwakiutl Indians, 2, 151

Lapps, 152
Leeches, 36, 37, 99
Leeuwenhoek, Anton van, 23
"Le Fort" operation, 131
LH (Luteinizing hormone), 27, 29
Libido, 120–121, 123, 140
    male compared to female, 119
Life expectancy, 4
Life span, human, 2–6
Lobus frontalis, 10
Lorenz, Konrad, 116

Mabaan tribe, 4
Malnutrition, 4, 144
Mammography, 136–137
Manbuti tribe, 116
Maori, 1
Mare, pregnant, 26
Marrow, 10
Masters, Dr. William H., 119
Maugham, W. Somerset, 2
Mead, Margaret, 16, 160
Mechanical Quackery, 157
Medical Letter, 66, 78
Memory lapses, 36, 57
Menopausal symptoms, 10–11, 18–
    20, 21, 29, 33–41, 54, 66, 67,
    71, 80, 99–100, 108, 117, 150
Menopause, 10–11, 11–12, 13, 26,
    46, 54, 55, 62, 70, 80–81, 89,
    91, 92–95, 101, 104, 116, 126,
    127, 134, 141, 159, 160
    early medical knowledge of, 17–
    20, 65, 121
    emotional reaction to, 16–17, 21–
    22, 29, 37–38, 56, 60, 67, 97,
    98, 100
    hormonal therapy for, 19–20, 21,
    51–64
    "Male," 122–124
    and middle age, 15–16, 20–22,
    150
    physiological changes in, 29–31
    "premature," 148–149
    prevention of, 71, 72, 147, 148
    surgical, 127, 128

188

Index

Menstruation, 15, 17, 24, 26–28, 29, 31, 35, 51, 53, 61, 62–63, 71, 93, 95, 101–110, 117, 128, 147–148, 149, 162
Mental health, 154
Merchants of Menace, The, 157
Mesmer, Friedrich Anton, 155
Metabolism theory of aging, 5
Metchnikoff, Élie, 8
Middle age, 15–16, 20–22, 28–31, 39, 89, 91, 92–95, 96, 122, 125, 150
  physical changes in, 73–88
Migraine, 99, 102, 140
  See also Headaches
Monilia, 114–115
Mongolian tribes, 151
Mozart, Wolfgang A., 89
Mucusless Diet Healing System, The, 82
Muslimov, Shirali, 2

National Health Council, 154
Nausea, 68–69
Navaho Indians, 8, 151
Nephritis, 131
Nerves, 74–75
"Neurohumors," 24
Never Too Late, 159
New Concept of Diagnosis and Treatment, 155
New Guinea tribes, 12
New York Public Health Department, 134
Niehans, Dr. Paul, 10–11
Night sweats, *see* Sweating
Norse mythology, 7
Novocaine, *see* Procaine

Obstetrics, 51, 162
Osteoarthritis, 40
Osteoporosis, 39, 64, 71, 143–147
Ovarian failure, complete, 149
Ovaries, 10, 18, 23, 25, 26, 27, 28, 29, 54, 71, 87, 117, 134, 148, 162
  cancer of, 48, 127, 134
  removal of, 28, 127–129, 139, 145
Overweight, 4, 79–83, 138, 141, 154
  See also Weight gaining

Ovulation, 28, 102–104, 106, 148–149, 161, 162

Pancreas, 25
"Pap" smear, 48, 57, 64, 97, 107, 133
Papanicolaou, Dr. George N., 51–52, 133
  See also "Pap" smear
Parathyroid, 10, 144
Patent medicines, 155
Payagua tribe, 84
Pelvic disorders, psychosomatic, 93
Perspiration rashes, 88
Pessary, 130
Physiotherapy, 41
Pickering, Sir George White, 7
Pigmentation, changes in, 30, 70
Pituitary gland, 6, 23–24, 26, 27, 28, 29, 34, 35, 76, 144, 148
  antidiuretic hormone, 102
  "ovary-stimulating" hormone, 27, 28, 162
"Pitcher's arm," 40
Placenta, 10, 26, 162
Plastic surgery:
  facial, 78–79
  breast, 86–88
Plato, 138, 160
Polygamy, 151
Polyps, 107, 108, 134
Ponce de León, Juan, 8
Population Council Laboratories, 114
Post-traumatic immobilization, 144
Posture problems, 88
Pregnancy, 16, 26–27, 45, 46, 52, 69, 70, 72, 73, 80, 104, 105, 106
  after menopause, 159–163
  fear of, 24, 116
Premenstrual tension syndrome, 101–105, 110
Procaine, 9
Progeria, 3
Progesterone, 25, 26, 27, 28, 29, 30, 45–46, 47, 48, 52, 61, 63, 69, 70, 71, 72, 86, 91, 102, 120, 149
Progestin, 49, 72, 85, 162
Prolapse:
  complete, 131

189